Improving Mental Health through Social Support

Building Positive and Empowering Relationships

Jonathan Leach

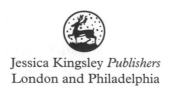

Jessica Kingsley *Publishers*
London and Philadelphia

First published in 2015
by Jessica Kingsley Publishers
73 Collier Street
London N1 9BE, UK
and
400 Market Street, Suite 400
Philadelphia, PA 19106, USA

www.jkp.com

Library of Congress Cataloging in Publication Data
Leach, Jonathan (Jonathan Stephen Roger)
Improving mental health through social support : building
positive and empowering relationships /
Jonathan Leach.
pages cm
Includes bibliographical references and index.
ISBN 978-1-84905-518-5 (alk. paper)
1. Mental health--Social aspects. 2. Social networks--
Health aspects. 3. Social networks--Psychological
aspects. 4. Mentally ill--Social networks. I. Title.
RA790.5.L33 2015
616.89--dc23
2014030709

British Library Cataloguing in Publication Data
A CIP catalogue record for this book is available from the British Library

ISBN 978 1 84905 518 5
eISBN 978 0 85700 932 6

Printed and bound in Great Britain by Bell and Bain Ltd, Glasgow

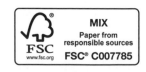

MIX
Paper from
responsible sources
FSC
www.fsc.org
FSC® C007785

'Jonathan Leach's clearly written book is an important contribution in helping us to understand the value of social support, its complex meanings, and how it can be provided in practice. It should be read by all mental health professionals.'

— Philip Thomas, former Consultant Psychiatrist, Bradford District Care Trust, and Honorary Visiting Professor, University of Bradford

'Getting the basics right about responding to people with a psychiatric diagnosis is vital. In this book Jonathan Leach makes the eminently sensible case that one of those needs is for human association. Social support reduces our risk of developing mental health problems and it increases our luck of recovery when and if they develop. A clear and well written case is made for the reader that social support not clever technologies should be a high priority in mental health policy.'

— David Pilgrim, Professor of Health and Social Policy, University of Liverpool

'Social support is essential for our mental health and must not be ignored in the rush towards psychological or pharmacological explanations for mental distress. This important book should be read by every health and social care student to ensure social perspectives are retained in our understanding of mental health.'

— Martin Webber, Director of the International Centre for Mental Health Social Research, University of York

Promoting Public Mental Health and Well-being
Principles into Practice
Jean S. Brown, Alyson M. Learmonth and Catherine J. Mackereth
Foreword by John R. Ashton
ISBN 978 1 84905 567 3
eISBN 978 1 78450 004 7

The Individual Service Funds Handbook
Implementing Personal Budgets in Provider Organisations
Helen Sanderson and Robin Miller
ISBN 978 1 84905 423 2
eISBN 978 0 85700 792 6

Mutual Support and Mental Health
A Route to Recovery
Maddy Loat
ISBN 978 1 84310 530 5
eISBN 978 0 85700 508 3
Community, Culture and Change series

Social Perspectives in Mental Health
Developing Social Models to Understand and Work with Mental Distress
Edited by Jerry Tew
Foreword by Judy Foster
ISBN 978 1 84310 220 5
eISBN 978 1 84642 102 0

The Equality Act 2010 in Mental Health
A Guide to Implementation and Issues for Practice
Edited by Hári Sewell
Foreword by Lord Victor Adebowale
ISBN 978 1 84905 284 9
eISBN 978 0 85700 589 2

Making Partnerships with Service Users and Advocacy Groups Work
How to Grow Genuine and Respectful Relationships in Health and Social Care
Julie Gosling and Jackie Martin
ISBN 978 1 84905 193 4
eISBN 978 0 85700 608 0

Reflective Practice in Mental Health
Advanced Psychosocial Practice with Children, Adolescents and Adults
Edited by Martin Webber and Jack Nathan
Foreword by Alan Rushton
ISBN 978 1 84905 029 6
eISBN 978 0 85700 396 6
Reflective Practice in Social Care series

Contents

Acknowledgements

I would like to thank: Kevin Harris and Liz Hodgson for reading and commenting on the first draft of this book; Joan Simons, my line manager at The Open University for encouraging and supporting me to take the time to get this book written; my colleague Mick McCormick for collaboration in producing the online survey of service users' attitudes that has fed into this work. I am also indebted to Mark Walsh who has offered valuable advice and support on the authoring process throughout the time I have been working on this book.

Preface

'Social support' refers to the everyday help and reassurance that friends, relatives, colleagues and others give each other throughout their lives. It can both protect against mental distress and help people cope with the effects of mental health problems. Unfortunately, the development of a mental health problem and the acquiring of a psychiatric diagnosis can lead to a diminution of social support for some individuals. Isolation is often associated with powerlessness, whereas positive connections with others can be empowering. The development of supportive networks is thus an important part of challenging social exclusion and discrimination. Although much has been written about medical and psychological approaches to supporting people with mental health problems, there is a surprising lack of similar coverage for social support. However, with the exception of the small percentage of service users being treated on hospital wards at any one time, the vast majority spend most of their time in the community rather than medical or psychotherapeutic settings.

Although writing this book took me around two years, the gestation period has been much longer. I joined a voluntary sector mental health organisation in the late 1980s, working alongside and teaching horticultural skills to people classed as having 'severe mental health problems'. This was at a time when the old long-stay psychiatric wards were being closed down and many of their former inhabitants were being placed 'in the community'. Having studied sociology in the 1970s, first as an A-level and then at degree level, I had encountered ideas about social control and how society categorises and labels those who are 'different'. However, this knowledge was not particularly useful in my daily interactions with the service users with whom I worked. With no background in nursing, social work, therapy, medicine or similar, I lacked a ready-made model of practice that might guide my work. Instead, as we worked side by side sowing seeds, potting up plants or preparing flower beds, I realised, first, that each person's medical diagnosis seemed to say very little about them and their capabilities; several people in the group were diagnosed as having 'schizophrenia' but they varied hugely in their motivation, behaviour and outlook on life. Other factors such as personality, life history, financial worries and current social situation appeared to have at least as much influence over their everyday lives. Second, I discovered how important it was for them to re-engage with everyday things like having a valued role, enjoying friendships, going to different places and making choices about what to buy or what to do. Long periods in hospital seemed to have reduced their ability to do many of these things that most of us probably take for granted.

I have a memory from about halfway through the ten years I spent working in the same organisation, of sitting in on a case review of one of the service users with whom I had worked closely. The psychiatrist, community psychiatric nurses and other professionals present spoke confidently about medication issues, care and treatment plans. I felt uncomfortable, as this discussion did not seem to reflect the breadth and depth of that individual's reality that I witnessed on a day-to-day basis. I also felt disempowered; they were professionals, who was I? I was not sure that I could impress them with my, by then, ten-year-old and relatively unused sociology degree. I had no professional status in a room where there was a clear hierarchy. I felt I had no voice in that situation, yet I probably knew the individual under review better than any of them. This sense of relative powerlessness led me to: study part-time for a master's degree in 'vocational rehabilitation and disability management at work'; become involved in, and for a period be chair of, the UK's Vocational Rehabilitation Association; and eventually move into academia to research and teach social aspects of mental health.

This book is influenced by, and draws on, those experiences of providing support that do not sit comfortably within a medical or psychotherapeutic paradigm yet appear to be very important for mental health. I have used ideas from sociology and allied subjects that seem to have a practical relevance for understanding the issues faced by people with mental health problems. However, this is not a sociology of mental health handbook. These already exist. Rather it is a sociologically informed exploration of the practical steps that can be taken by a range of people in both formal and informal roles to provide everyday support to individuals and groups who have been disadvantaged through their experience of mental health problems.

Increasingly, mental health policy is shifting its focus of attention towards community care, personalisation and social inclusion. This creates a need to promote understanding of the practicalities of everyday support by friends, relatives and others operating in a non-professional or informal capacity. Mental health and social care professionals will need a more sophisticated understanding of the dynamics of social support in order to work effectively with service users in the community. Providers of support from voluntary sector agencies are being expected to deliver a range of community services and to provide evidence to their funders of the quality of the support they offer, which is largely social in nature. Service users and carers are increasingly looking at models of mutual support and empowerment to guide their actions. The concept of social support provides a useful theoretical and practical foundation upon which to develop these models.

Some books have been written on the possible social causes of mental health problems and on the links between social capital and mental health, but very little has been written on what social support means in practice. This book's major focus is the nature of interactions between service users and their supporters and carers in a range of contexts. It will be of interest to people working in the voluntary sector and community-based services, social workers, mental health professionals and others who are interested in working across the boundaries of service provision and everyday life. It will also provide useful insights for those studying and teaching on social work, health and social care courses. Service users and those who provide informal support to them should also find much of interest.

Starting with the lessons that can be learnt from the fields of sociology and allied disciplines, some barriers and some possible solutions to obtaining social support for people with mental health problems are explored. The nature of this support is examined both in informal settings, such as friendship groups, families and communities, and in more formal contexts, such as educational institutions and workplaces. The book concludes by looking at the broader perspective of social support within communities and how such support can be fostered.

Chapter 1

A friend in need

Rediscovering social support

Introduction

Most people experience a degree of mental distress at some point, but only a relatively small proportion will seek professional help. This means that many individuals are likely to derive informal social support from friends and family. If such support is not available, or not sufficient for their needs, some will seek or be directed towards medical or psychotherapeutic services. Even so, with the exception of the relatively low number of people who are currently hospital inpatients, most mental health service users will spend the majority of their time in the community. Whether or not that community has a positive influence on their mental health will depend on a number of factors, including the amount of social support that is available. In turn, the support offered by members of a community will be influenced by how they view 'mental health' and 'mental distress' and whether or not they feel they can offer meaningful and effective help.

Concepts of mental health and distress

Whenever mental health is mentioned, it is often, in fact, the opposite that is being referred to. For instance, by far the greatest proportion of resources allocated to 'mental health services' are devoted to helping to control the symptoms of mental ill-health of individuals whose condition is considered serious enough to warrant professional services. By contrast, relatively little expenditure is allocated to promote the mental health of the general population or to analyse and address the social conditions that might cause mental distress. This is not to deny that mental health professionals try to improve quality of life for those who use their services, but rather to suggest that there is often a stronger policy focus on responding to things that go wrong in individuals' lives instead of considering what makes them go well. The recent expansion of interest in 'positive psychology', both in the academic literature and in the wider market for books on self-help and self-improvement, may seem to be redressing the balance, but as yet it is not clear whether this will have any impact on the practice of mental health and social work services or on wider social policy.

Mental health is a slippery concept and perhaps not one that most people tend to pay as much attention to as physical health (Jorm 2000). No definition is perfect, and it is difficult to avoid cultural assumptions. Nevertheless, it is important to be at least reasonably clear about what is meant when one uses the term. I tend to see mental health as a collection of abilities:

- An awareness both of one's surrounding in the physical and social environments and how one interacts with those environments.

- The ability to make choices and to set goals by realistically appraising one's own capacities in relation to the surrounding environment.

- The ability to relate to others in a culturally appropriate manner and to enjoy at least some of those relationships.

- The ability to respond emotionally to positive or negative situations and return to a less emotional state over time.

In these terms, mental health is not simply about feeling happy or sad. A person could be manically happy whilst behaving in a highly extravagant and risky fashion with little regard for others. If this continues for a lengthy period it could be difficult to argue that it is a healthy situation. Conversely, there are events, such as bereavement, job loss and relationship breakdown, where at least in the short term, sadness is an appropriate and healthy response. So, rather than being happy all the time, mental health is more about having some control over the direction of one's feelings, thoughts and actions, even though this will be disrupted from time to time by various challenges.

In this book I will discuss how social support can enhance mental health for all, whilst paying particular attention to how that support might be targeted at those people who, through experiences of mental ill-health or distress, have become socially isolated, excluded and vulnerable. Deciding what terminology to use for such problematic experiences can be difficult. I have already used the term 'mental ill-health' twice in this chapter, but does this mean that experiences that have been labelled with terms such as depression, anxiety, phobia, anorexia, bipolar disorder or schizophrenia can be considered to be illnesses similar to ailments such as asthma, diabetes and heart disease? There is a bio-medical view that these and other similar mental conditions are all 'illnesses' and should be treated as such, even if as yet there are no reliable physical tests for confirming their presence. Here, terms such as 'mental illness' or 'psychiatric disorder' may be used to cover such conditions (Gelder, Mayou and Geddes 2005). Another view is that the experiences classed as 'psychoses', chiefly schizophrenia and bipolar disorder, are disorders with a biological basis, but those classed as 'neuroses', including anxiety and depression, are more likely to arise as understandable responses to negative life events (Jorm 2000).

To some extent, a social support perspective can take a neutral stance on what the root causes of mental health problems are, as the main focus is on what practical and emotional help to offer. However, causation is a contentious issue in the mental health field. Some writers, for example Richard Bentall (2010) and Lucy Johnstone (2009), question the very notion of mental 'illness' and argue that the types of conditions mentioned can all be understood in psychological or social terms without reference to bio-medical explanations. I have explored these conflicting approaches elsewhere (Leach 2009) but mention them here to illustrate the difficulties in finding a language to use that is not tied to one explanatory framework. The term 'patient' is very firmly tied to a medical framework and so does not relate to people who are not currently being treated by a health professional. Similarly, words such as 'lunatic' and 'mad', although now embraced by some people with mental health problems, are loaded with derogatory meaning for many people. In this book I will tend to use the terms 'distress', 'disturbance' or 'problems' to refer to the experiences of people who are having difficulties with their mental health, whilst accepting that even this is less than perfect. For instance, some people may hear voices but not be distressed about them. In some instances, particularly when discussing how psychiatry categorises people, I will use the term 'disorder', as this reflects the experience of a significant proportion of distressed people who receive a clinical diagnosis. I have tended to use the term 'service user' in this book as a shorthand way of referring to people who have been in contact with mental health services and more generally will refer to 'people with mental health problems' whilst leaving open the question of whether these 'problems' are caused by social, psychological or biological factors.

The example of hearing voices without being distressed by them raises a question: can someone who has been diagnosed by a mental health professional as having a 'psychiatric disorder' or 'mental illness', such as schizophrenia, still experience 'mental health'? The concept of two continua, one for mental health and one for mental disorder (Tudor 1996), could be helpful here, although, as will be discussed in the next chapter, this is only one of a number of ways that the subject can be conceptualised. A mental disorder continuum would have severe symptoms of a diagnosed (or potentially diagnosable) disorder at the higher end and the absence of such symptoms at the lower end. A mental health continuum would place feelings of extreme mental distress and unhappiness at the lower end and feelings of well-being at the top. Looking back at the mental health abilities listed earlier in this section, it can be seen that each of these can also be represented as a continuum. For instance, some people are better able to form and enjoy social relationships than others.

Positions on the mental health and mental disorder continua are linked but not necessarily in a rigid fashion. Although high levels of mental disorder are typically linked to low levels of mental health, this does not apply universally. Many people who would not be diagnosed as having a psychiatric disorder (lower end of the mental disorder continuum) will have periods in their lives when they are very distressed and unhappy (lower end of the mental health continuum). People who have been diagnosed as having schizophrenia, bipolar disorder and other psychiatric disorders (higher end of the mental disorder continuum) can, in the right circumstances, experience feelings of well-being and happiness in their lives (higher end of the mental health continuum). Those experiencing conditions such as depression and anxiety are likely to be at the higher end of the mental disorder continuum and at the lower end of the mental health continuum. Whatever the diagnosed condition, helping distressed individuals to move from the lower to the higher end of the mental health continuum would seem to be a worthwhile goal and one that can be assisted through supportive relationships.

Social support

'Social support' is used in this book to refer to various forms of help encountered within the environments in which people live, work, study and play. Some aspects of social support, such as establishing a caring relationship, helping to give meaning to distress and attempting to promote change, may share features with formal psychological support (Barker and Pistrang 2002). However, social support differs in being less structured and more likely to occur in everyday contexts. Often informal in nature, social support arises out of the network of friends, family and acquaintances, such as neighbours and work colleagues, surrounding an individual.

Social support is important to both physical and mental health. Lack of social support is associated with social isolation and feelings of loneliness. A survey by Mind (2004) reported that 84 per cent of respondents who had used mental health services in the UK felt isolated. This contrasted with 29 per cent of the general population who identified themselves as isolated. Even when a person has a 'social network' of people they know, they can feel lonely if those relationships are unsupportive or, worse still, actually detrimental to their well-being (Segrin and Passalacqua 2010). Social support is not simply a matter of how many people you know, but also how supportive they are towards you. Loneliness has been associated with poorer physical health and reduced life expectancy, particularly in relation to an increased risk of cardiovascular problems (Hawkley and Cacioppo 2010). Similarly, feelings of loneliness have been associated with an increased risk of a wide range of cognitive and mental health problems (Hawkley and Cacioppo 2010). The absence of close, confiding relationships has been found to be a significant factor in predicting depression and anxiety (Harrison et al. 1999). Although there can clearly be a two-way relationship between loneliness and mental distress, a review of the research indicates that conditions such as depression can be predicted by prior experiences of loneliness (Cacioppo, Hawkley and Thisted 2010).

A factor affecting the likelihood of informal social support being offered to someone experiencing mental distress is the attitude taken to mental health problems by those around them. Various surveys have examined the 'social distance' that respondents would put between themselves and someone known to have a mental health condition. In England the Office for National Statistics has commissioned research on this topic in an attempt to track changes in attitudes over a number of years. A recent report in this series painted a fairly positive picture in that 84 per cent of respondents agreed that no one should be excluded from their neighbourhood on the basis of having a 'mental illness', and 80 per cent agreed that being part of a normal community would be the best therapy for many people with mental illness (Prior 2010). However, such reports need to be treated with caution, as they measure what people say they believe rather than what they do in practice. Less acceptance might be found at a more personal level. For instance, only 26 per cent of respondents felt that a woman who had in the past been treated in a mental hospital could be trusted to carry out babysitting (Prior 2010). An analysis of surveys of 'social distance' in relation to mental health problems across a range of countries found that the greatest distance was desired in relation to people with substance abuse problems, followed by schizophrenia and then depression (Jorm and Oh 2009). The same authors were critical of the lack of research into people's behaviour rather than merely the attitudes they expressed to a researcher.

Whatever attitudes surveys tell us, there is no doubt that many people are affected by the actual or potential stigma (a concept explored in the next chapter) associated with mental health problems. A survey of over 3000 UK mental health service users reported that stigma had a negative effect on the lives of 87 per cent of respondents, and 73 per cent indicated that they had stopped doing various activities because of fear of stigma (Corry 2008). The impact of this stigma reduces the opportunities for people experiencing mental health problems to build networks of social support and increases their risk of social exclusion and isolation.

The 1980s saw a strong interest, particularly amongst American social scientists, in the role of social support in society. Working in the field of communication studies, Terrance Albrecht and Mara Adelman (1987) argued that there are three main aspects to social support interactions. First, they meet a need for human contact, which involves making sense of one's life and the events that occur within it. Second, a supportive interaction helps to reduce feelings of uncertainty, both about the situation the person finds themselves living in and about their relationship with the other person. This leads to the individual having a greater sense of control over their life and over the stressful conditions that might adversely affect them. Finally, social support takes place within a structure of connected and reciprocal relationships, some strong and some weak, in which help is given and received. Although these authors were examining social support in the context of the general population, the three aspects they identified seem to have particular relevance for improving mental health and reducing the impact of mental distress.

The UK has also seen interest in understanding social support. Social psychologist Michael Argyle and colleagues (Argyle, Bryant and Trower 1974) identified the importance of social support for general well-being but also suggested that social skills training could play a major role in mental health treatment. Similarly, sociologists George Brown and Tirril Harris undertook groundbreaking work on the role of social support in reducing the risk of depression (Brown *et al.* 1986) and positively evaluated the benefits of befriending as an intervention for depression (Harris, Brown and Robinson 1999). Graham Allan (1989, 2008) has taken a sociological approach to exploring the impact of friendship and kinship. Allan suggests that, beyond the companionship and sociability that accompanies friendship, there can be a high level of personal support including emotional, moral and practical support. Clinical psychologist Derek Milne (1999), studying the support given by friends and others encountered informally (e.g. hairdressers), identified a similar range of benefits and suggested that health professionals could foster such support in communities to improve the well-being of mental health service users. User-led research has also found that both emotional and practical support are valued by mental health service users when engaging with everyday difficulties (Faulkner and Layzell 2000).

More recently, American sociologists R. Jay Turner and Robyn Brown (2010) have referred to social support as a multidimensional construct comprising: perceived support, structural support and received support. These two authors suggest that *perceived support* (knowing that support is available should one need it) provides two main benefits: protecting the individual from the effects of stressful factors and enabling their personal and social development. *Structural support* refers to the framework of social ties and networks that the individual is part of and which acts as a resource for them. This is similar to the notion of 'social capital' (Putnam 2000), which implies the presence of reciprocal relationships. In other words, both parties feel that that they have something to gain from each other. *Received support* consists of the actual provision of helpful information or practical assistance provided by others.

It would seem that social support can play an important part in everyday life, helping people to feel connected with each other, have a valued identity and be better able to deal with stressful conditions. This could be described as a 'virtuous circle' in that being able to call on social support improves well-being, which in turn makes it easier to engage with other people and build more and deeper supportive relationships. By contrast, when mental distress is particularly severe and long-lasting, there is a distinct danger of a 'downward spiral' whereby the person affected does not feel like socialising, is less able to reciprocate any support received and may start to lose a number of relationships. This in turn could make them feel more depressed, anxious and distrustful and less able to cope with stressful situations, leading to a further loss of socially supportive relationships.

A historical view

What can we learn about social support from history? Was there ever a golden age when most people lived in supportive communities that cared for their mentally distressed members, or does history show that such people were amongst the outcasts of society? This is not an easy question to answer, particularly as definitions of 'madness' or 'lunacy' (terms used much more in the past than the present) are loose and changeable over time. Not many of the numerous 'disorders' that are now listed in the diagnostic manuals used by psychiatrists would have been recognised as such in the past. It is likely that only the most severe and dramatic incidences of mental distress would have been recorded in historical sources.

Social historian Roy Porter (2002) suggests that across Europe from the classical era to the Middle Ages it was the family who were expected to deal with their disturbed relatives. In some instances they were confined within the home; in others they were sent away to wander and survive as best they could by begging and relying on charity. If the types of behaviour we would now associate with severe cases of schizophrenia and bipolar disorder were then explained in terms of possession by demons or degenerate breeding, families would have been deeply ashamed and stigmatised by having a member seen as being 'mad'. This would have made it very difficult for distressed and disturbed individuals to become integrated within local communities. In the Middle Ages, charitable religious institutions started providing care for some of the most dispossessed and disturbed people in European societies. In England, the best-known lunatic asylum, 'Bedlam', arose out of the London-based religious institution St Mary of Bethlehem founded in 1247 (Porter 2002). In the following centuries, further charitable and private asylums developed across the UK and Europe, and these institutions gained powers to confine a wide range of people who did not fit with society's norms (Foucault 1965).

According to the researches of another social historian, Andrew Scull (1989), the inmates of asylums were widely regarded as dangerous and sub-human creatures who needed to be chained up and subject to all kinds of physical torments in order to keep their wild natures under control. Sadly, in the past it was regarded as popular entertainment to go and view the 'lunatics' and people visited Bedlam as one of the sights of London, in the manner of a circus freak show (Porter 2002). In contrast to this cruel and degrading treatment, a more benign approach was developed in the 18th century in the form of what became known as 'moral treatment'.

Moral treatment was developed by pioneers such as Philippe Pinel in France and William Tuke in England; it was exemplified in the Quaker institution the York Retreat founded in 1796 (Borthwick et al. 2001). In the Retreat, the use of chains and violence on patients was forbidden. Instead, patients were provided with a pleasant environment, wholesome food, practical roles and duties to perform. Importantly, they were encouraged to form social relationships with staff, fellow patients and visitors drawn largely from the local Quaker community. This is an early example of formalised social support in which it was believed that treating and interacting with patients in a positive manner would raise their morale and self-esteem, which in turn would reduce their mental distress.

In the UK, there was no significant state intervention in the treatment of mental distress until the 19th century. In England, public funding for treatment in asylums was legislated for in 1808 and in 1844 English counties were required to provide asylums. Over this century, there was a tenfold increase in the number of patients in English asylums (Porter 2002). This growth, first of private asylums and subsequently public institutions, provided the context within which the profession of psychiatry was to develop. In any era, the challenge for informal social supporters, such as family, friends and neighbours, is to know to whom to turn when their help no longer seems to be sufficient for the person concerned. From the accounts of social historians (which tend to focus on those people with the most severe problems) it would seem that, for many, the only help provided was to lock the disturbed person away in an asylum.

The idea that 'madness' could be treated by medical practitioners started to take hold in the 19th century. The term 'psychiatry' was first used in British medicine in 1846 (Rogers and Pilgrim 2001). In 1841, the forerunner of the Royal College of Psychiatrists was formed as the Association of Medical Officers of Asylums and Hospitals for the Insane. Similarly, in the USA, 1844 saw the establishment of the Association of Medical Superintendents of American Institutions for the Insane, which later developed into the American Psychiatric Association (Porter 2002). In Germany, the discipline of psychiatry grew through the work of Emil Kraepelin (1856–1926) who started to develop a diagnostic system for what we now term 'psychoses' that could be used by practitioners in different countries (Bentall 2010).

At the same point in history, Sigmund Freud (1856–1939) working in the emerging field of psychology promoted an interest in the study of the causes and treatment of 'neuroses' (Burns 2006). At first this interest manifested itself in the offering of private individual psychotherapy to the relatively few patients who could afford the frequent therapy sessions required by the psychoanalytic approach. However, the impetus for taking 'neurotic' conditions more seriously seems to have come from the experience of medical practitioners being faced with formerly healthy young men who returned from the battlefield of the First World War with 'shellshock'. According to sociologists Anne Rogers and David Pilgrim (2001), this had a number of consequences, including: moving the scope of professional interest from psychosis to include neurosis, a realisation that environmental factors could cause mental health problems and the extension of medical services from inpatient to outpatient provision. This paved the way for offering professional support for a wider range of mental conditions than those formerly encountered within the asylum system.

The professionalisation of mental health support

The sympathy, understanding and support given to anyone experiencing mental distress is likely to be affected by commonly held views in the wider population about what causes mental health problems. Mediaeval ideas of madness caused by demonic possession led to fear and social distancing. By contrast, it would be hoped that biological and psychological explanations could improve matters. In line with this approach, the idea of educating the public that mental health problems are an illness that can be treated by a doctor, like any other illness, could be seen as an effective means of reducing stigma and increasing understanding.

Emphasising genetic factors in causation is one way in which mental health problems are presented as an illness. Proponents of this view point to the tendency for certain mental disorders to run through families. Explanations of a genetic basis for mental health conditions might seem to enable them to be viewed more rationally and positively. This hope has been challenged both on theoretical grounds (Phelan 2002) and in the research literature (Read, Mosher and Bentall 2004). One reason for these challenges is that describing someone with, for example, a diagnosis of schizophrenia, as biologically and genetically distinct from other people can lead to them being more strongly labelled as 'other'. If they are viewed as having defective genes, this threatens their potential to be accepted into intimate relationships because of the risk of any future offspring inheriting such genes. The genetic causal explanation also implies that the person will never be free of their diagnosis, making it a very 'sticky label' throughout their life.

Another hope in promoting a genetic or illness model could be that it would reduce the possibility of parents being blamed for causing their children's mental health problems through faulty upbringing or

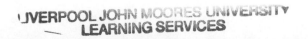

unhealthy patterns of interactions. Although this might be the case, an additional problem arises in that the whole family might attract stigma as carriers of 'faulty genes' (Phelan 2002). The role of the family has long been a difficult area in the history of mental health. Clearly, 'blaming' a person's family is not conducive to maintaining a good working relationship with professionals nor to helping relatives support a distressed individual. Nevertheless, the psychodynamic tradition tends to see early experiences within the family as highly significant contributors to 'neurotic' conditions. And while subsequent writers might not attribute blame, as radical psychiatrists R.D. Laing and Aaron Esterson (1970) were seen to do in the 1960s and 1970s, proponents of a socially informed psychological approach such as Lucy Johnstone (2000), John Read *et al.* (2004) and Richard Bentall (2010), all consider that the family plays a role in the development of 'psychotic' conditions.

Common or 'lay' perceptions of the causes of mental health problems make it likely that many families will feel 'responsible', at least in part, for any mental health conditions experienced by their offspring. Compared with the views of medical professionals, lay understandings of mental health tend to place greater emphasis on stressful situations in an individual's life as causal factors in the development of both neurotic and psychotic conditions (Jorm 2000). Because family, past and present, features strongly in many people's lives, family relationships can be put under the spotlight at times of personal breakdown: 'Where did we go wrong?' This is relevant to social support because families can be a major source of support to their distressed members, but if relationships are strained this support may be weakened. There is also the question of whether it can be assumed that support from family members will always be sufficient or suitable for an individual's well-being. The role of the family is examined later in this book.

When family or friends can no longer provide all the support the individual needs this can act as a trigger to accessing help from a professional. The first port of call is often the general practitioner (GP). A survey on attitudes to mental health service usage in the UK conducted by The Open University found that 89 per cent of respondents first approached their GP; a typical response being: 'Who else?' (The Open University 2011). If the GP assesses the person's need as great enough they will refer them on to a psychiatrist or other mental health specialist. However, gaining access to specialised professional support could be a mixed blessing for the individual in terms of on-going social support. Extreme and prolonged mental distress can leave those close to the person feeling anxious and helpless, in which case it could be reassuring to know that professional care is available. For the person affected it can also be a relief that their problems are being taken seriously and are identified as a recognisable condition than can be treated. However, the fact that someone is seen as so disturbed that they need specialist professional interventions could put them into a social category of people to be avoided and feared (Summerfield 2001).

The most severe incidences of mental distress and disturbance can have such obvious outward signs and symptoms that, if the person does not seek treatment themselves, others are likely to encourage them to do so. In the more extreme instances, individuals can be admitted to psychiatric institutions for treatment against their own wishes. However, for the majority of people their mental distress is less dramatic and they have to weigh up the pros and cons of talking about their experiences with others, whether that is friends and family or a health professional. A particularly influential piece of work on the numbers of people who do and don't seek or receive treatment was carried out in the UK in the 1980s and 1990s by psychiatrists David Goldberg and Peter Huxley (1992). They compared the number of people indicated by community surveys to be experiencing mental distress serious enough to benefit from professional intervention with the numbers presenting for and recognised as needing treatment. The focus was on 'common mental disorders', chiefly anxiety and depression and, according to their findings, up to 315 people in every thousand suffered significant mental distress affecting them for at least four weeks within the period of one year. Of these, 230 attended primary care, but just over 100 had their condition recognised by a GP. Around 23 people went on to use specialist mental health services.

More recently a household survey in England (McManus *et al.* 2009) found that, during the week previous to being interviewed, just over 15 per cent of respondents had symptoms indicating a 'common mental disorder'. Half of these respondents had symptoms severe enough for treatment to be required, but only 32 per cent of this group were actually receiving treatment. In the other half with symptoms that were not considered severe enough to require treatment, 17 per cent were in receipt of treatment. This leaves a lot of distressed people who, if they do not receive social support, will have no support at all. The same survey reported that for 'psychotic' disorders, the likely incidence over the past year was 0.4 per cent of respondents, of whom 81 per cent were receiving treatment. A previous national survey found that those with the most severe neurotic symptoms were the least likely to seek help from a GP. The two most common reasons for not seeking help were: 'did not think anyone could help' and 'a problem one should be able to cope with' (Meltzer *et al.* 2000, p.323).

An individual's self-perception is likely to change if they become someone who requires professional treatment. Researcher Kristian Pollock (2007) describes how people experiencing depression were concerned to maintain 'face' in social and medical encounters. Fears that others would see them as weak and inadequate and wouldn't understand them led to depressed respondents trying to conceal the problem in social encounters. In medical consultations, even though the individual attended with the intention of seeking help, the need to maintain face often prevented them from revealing their true feelings. Another piece of research (Cornford, Hill and Reilly 2007) found that patients' views of their depressive symptoms were quite different from those of mainstream medical practitioners. These patients were more likely to see their problems arising from a series of setbacks in life rather than being an illness. Although they did not rule out the benefits of medication, this was seen as only one aspect of managing their condition. Support from family and friends, as well as professionals, was seen as important. In addition, they were likely to favour a strategy of making themselves engage with social events and other activities in order to try and move beyond their depressed self that would rather withdraw from interaction with others.

Medical practitioners themselves are aware of the difficulties of distinguishing between normal reactions to life events, or difficult circumstances, and what could be regarded as 'psychiatric disorders'. To some extent, the fact that a significant number of patients are feeling depressed but are not diagnosed as such may reflect not only patients' reluctance to disclose their condition but also GPs' feelings that it could be unhelpful to give their patients' experiences a medical label (Rait *et al.* 2009). Guidelines on the treatment of depression in the UK recommend a period of 'watchful waiting' before considering the prescription of antidepressants, unless the condition is severe (National Institute for Health and Clinical Excellence 2009). This reflects the experience that some people get better without medical intervention. Although social support is recommended as part of a stepped-care approach to depression in primary care (Haddad *et al.* 2008), it is not clear how primary care practitioners could enable this for their patients. In contrast, it is relatively easy to write a prescription for medication or to make a referral for counselling, although in the case of the latter, waiting times and costs may be an issue.

Psychiatry, community care and social support

From the previous discussion it is clear that only a relatively small proportion of the people who experience mental distress or disturbance will come under specialist psychiatric rather than primary care. However, for those who do, there can be particular challenges in relation to social support, especially when a period of inpatient treatment is required. Conditions such as schizophrenia and bipolar disorder are more likely to result in periods of inpatient treatment in a mental hospital, and there is a greater stigma attached to the label of schizophrenia than there is to that of some other conditions such as depression (Corry 2008). A diagnosis of personality disorder can also be very stigmatising (Wright, Haigh and McKeeown 2009). People with mental health problems have reported how former friends drifted out of contact once they were in hospital, making it more likely that most of their relationships were with other service users rather than with a wider section of the community (Green *et al.* 2002).

The fact that people can be detained or treated against their wishes under mental health legislation adds a particular edge to being known as a psychiatric patient and to taking the decision to approach health services for help with mental distress. In the popular mind, mental health institutions may have become associated with the containment of individuals whom others find strange, disturbing and threatening. The separation of mental patients from the community that began on a large scale with the old Victorian asylums continued into the 20th century. Although initial proposals were made to introduce some level of community treatment and civil rights for people with mental health problems in the UK, legislation enacted in 1930 maintained a containment approach (Rogers and Pilgrim 2001). Power to detain patients was given to medical practitioners without the need to involve the judicial system. However, after the Second World War there was a loss of faith in the old asylums. A series of scandals about the mistreatment of long-stay patients, combined with ideological opposition to the containment approach and other factors, led to a change in policy. By 1954, UK inpatient numbers had reached a peak of 150,000 but during the early 1990s were reduced to around 50,000 (Rogers and Pilgrim 2001). The pace of change quickened in the 1980s, when the concept of 'care in the community' was promoted by policy makers.

One key concern about the old long-stay mental hospitals was the tendency for patients, and to some extent staff, to become 'institutionalised'. The effects of institutionalisation were highlighted by the work of American sociologist Erving Goffman with the publication of his book *Asylums* in 1961. Here, Goffman demonstrated that whatever issues brought people into mental institutions, the rigid and depersonalising procedures they encountered there caused a whole set of new problems for them. In adopting the persona of 'patient', the individual seemed to lose the social skills and confidence needed to live in the community. Now that service users tend to spend shorter periods of time in hospital, and smaller inpatient units have tried to become less like the 'total institutions' described by Goffman in the 1960s, it might be assumed that the problem has been solved. In practice, some level of institutionalisation can still be a risk, even in small inpatient units and community-based services.

It would be hoped that a system of community care for mental distress could lead to better integration and more social support with less need for dependence on the input of professionals. In the UK, there have certainly been improvements as a result of community care, but the changes have not been as far-reaching as might have been expected. Despite the involvement of the voluntary sector in service delivery, the way that community care was enacted still placed considerable emphasis on, and thus funding for, hospital psychiatry (Rogers and Pilgrim 2001). Although multidisciplinary community-based mental health teams have been set up, there have been concerns about some former patients ending up in poor living conditions with little support, affected by lack of funding and reflecting a failure of 'care in the community' (Hannigan and Coffey 2011). A medical-psychiatric model of mental health treatment still seems to dominate community care (Colombo *et al.* 2003), which, it could be argued, would benefit from being informed more strongly by a social perspective (Tew *et al.* 2012).

A common aspect of a psychiatric model of treatment is the prescription of medication for mental health problems. Over and above the effects of severe mental distress and disturbance themselves, the side effects of medication for long-term mental conditions may affect the service user's ability to access social support. Despite changes in the nature of medication available, there are concerns about side effects such as lethargy, loss of sexual interest and difficulties in maintaining concentration (Moncrieff 2009). All of these effects can have an impact on the individual's ability to make and sustain relationships and may perpetuate the views of others about them being different to 'normal' people.

The issues of compulsory treatment and widespread use of psychiatric medication have been taken up by service user movements, some of whom describe themselves as 'survivors' of the mental health system. User movements have challenged institutional approaches to treating mental distress and have campaigned on issues of civil rights and consumer choice. They have succeeded in securing representation on advisory and management bodies in the mental health sector, where they may have some influence if not power (Beresford 2009). Service-user-led organisations have also developed self-help groups, for example to support people who hear voices or who are depressed. Similarly, carers' and relatives' organisations have tried to influence mental health policy and practice and, in some cases, have become involved in providing services; such groups can be seen as a semi-formalised form of social support.

Conclusion: recognising social support

The topics of mental health and distress provoke a lively debate about probable causes, suitable terminology, appropriate treatment and issues of power and control. Although some writers have argued for social explanations of mental distress and disturbance as an alternative to medical and psychological models, social support neither confirms nor contradicts bio-medical or psychological approaches. Social support can co-exist with psychiatric and psychological treatments; indeed it can be argued that it is an essential ingredient in any package of measures designed to tackle mental health problems. This book does not assume that social support is all that is needed to improve mental health, but it promotes the idea that mental well-being is enhanced by appropriate social support and that medical and psychological interventions alone are unlikely to sustain recovery from mental distress.

Compared with previous eras, there are now many more conditions that could be considered to fall within the scope of the mental health professions. Attitudes may have moved on since the days of explaining madness as a sign of demonic possession, but issues of stigma and discrimination still figure as problems for people with mental health problems. The resulting isolation can only exacerbate any existing problems and act as an obstacle to recovery. Social support has many valuable features that can promote the well-being of vulnerable people, and this tends to be situated in the natural settings of home, workplace and community rather than in a clinical environment.

Chapter 2

Social aspects of mental health and distress

Introduction

The American sociologist C. Wright Mills suggested that one of the key roles of the sociologist is to illuminate how seemingly private troubles are actually public issues (Mills 1970). For instance, in the late 19th century, Emile Durkheim realised that something as apparently personal and individual as suicide, when looked at in terms of the levels of incidence in different countries and social groups, seems to be influenced by the type of society in which the person lives (Durkheim 1971, first published 1897). In contrast to psychological understandings of friendship, social interactions and mental distress, which focus on the characteristics of the individual, sociology looks at the wider social contexts within which that individual operates. This chapter will explore some of the theories that attempt to explain issues of mental distress, identity and relationships and the impact of social contexts on mental health.

Understanding mental health problems

In the previous chapter, it was suggested that mental health problems can be understood from a number of perspectives including the bio-medical, psychological and social. This chapter focuses on theories that inform social perspectives, as these are particularly relevant to the exploration of social support for mental health. A broad range of social and sociological theories suggest that what might at first seem to be individual and personal problems can also be understood within a social context.

Friendships tend to be made when people identify themselves as similar in various significant ways (Allan 1989). So when considering the need for social support, it is useful to examine whether having a 'mental disorder' can be distinguished from the commonly experienced problems of distress and unhappiness in life. If there is a distinction, it could mean that people labelled as 'disordered' are seen as different in some important sense by those around them. In this case, there might need to be an extra dimension to the support offered to people who have a diagnosed disorder, over and above what one friend might do for another during difficult times. The idea of two continua, one for mental disorder and one for mental health, has already been proposed in Chapter 1. Acceptance of this duality would indicate that it is possible to separate the everyday ups and downs of life from those mental disorders that have a much longer-term impact on an individual's ability to cope. An alternative explanation is that there is only one continuum, with mental health (typically represented by absence of diagnosable disorders) at one end and mental ill-health (presence of diagnosable disorders) at the other. At the risk of complicating matters further, an American sociologist Andrew Payton (2009) suggests that, instead, we should be considering the existence of three distinct continua: distress, disorder and mental health.

Payton starts by reviewing the concepts used by sociologists when writing about distress, disorder and mental health. He then looks for evidence for these being distinct or overlapping phenomena by examining survey research findings on a large adult sample in the USA population. In this analysis, *distress* is measured by statements about unpleasant feelings, *disorder* by the presence of symptoms that would be used to make a psychiatric diagnosis and *mental health* relates to looking at what makes people flourish and feel content, the latter being the subject area of interest to positive psychologists. Payton judged all three concepts to be distinct phenomena, although, not surprisingly, found that they are related to each other. If these are different phenomena then it suggests that sociology and other related disciplines should be careful to specify what they are investigating when addressing issues that have typically come under the umbrella term of 'mental health'.

The concepts suggested by Payton can be illustrated by imagining the case of a man who has been diagnosed with the mental *disorder* of schizophrenia, the main feature of which is hearing several critical voices. His levels of mental *distress*, such as fear, anger and despair, vary according to the experience of hearing the voices and what they are saying at any one time, but are also affected by how other people react to him. His *mental health* is currently limited by his difficulty in focusing on forming and pursuing meaningful personal goals and in forming close relationships. This separation of the man's difficulties into three conceptual areas then suggests different supportive interventions for each. The impact of the voices might be addressed by medication, self-help techniques or attending a support group for voice-hearers. His feelings of distress might be helped by talking therapies, relaxation techniques or engagement with others in social activities. His mental health might be promoted by coaching and mentoring to find meaningful personal goals and by the provision of training and support to develop his social skills. Improvement in any one area may have a positive impact on the others and the best outcomes are likely to be achieved by addressing all three. In this analysis, a role for bio-medicine or psychotherapy is not ruled out, but it can be seen that socially supportive interventions could play an important part.

Payton's ideas, although interesting and potentially useful, do not adequately answer the question of how distress can reliably be distinguished from disorder. He takes the Diagnostic and Statistical Manual of Mental Disorders (DSM) of the American Psychiatric Association as a reference point for identifying disorder, but this shifts the question to how use of the DSM or a similar instrument distinguishes distress from disorder. On a simple level, mental disorder is whatever is labelled as such by a psychiatrist or other relevant professional using recognised diagnostic criteria. British clinical psychologist Derek Bolton (2010) points out that these diagnostic criteria do not occur in isolation, but rather reflect thinking in the wider society. In his view, a necessary condition for identifying mental disorder is the presence of personally unmanageable distress that disrupts an individual's daily activities; in other words, the extent to which the person becomes disabled is a key factor. This is what is likely to trigger an appointment with a health professional in the first place. Bolton proposes that, following on from this initial contact, the professional and the patient negotiate the meaning of the problems experienced, thus deciding whether and how to define those problems as a health issue. The diagnostic criteria set out in psychiatric handbooks are used as part of that negotiation process, with the professional asking the patient a series of questions designed to match their experiences to recognised disorders.

Although the use of diagnostic tools can be seen as bringing objectivity to the process, American sociologist Jerome Wakefield (2010) argues that psychiatric diagnostic guidelines, such as the DSM, have difficulty in distinguishing normal variations in human feelings from disorders. Even though the DSM takes into account events such as bereavement, Wakefield feels that the way the current diagnostic criteria are set out makes them quite capable of pathologising normal distress. For instance, extreme symptoms of normal sadness, caused by a relationship break-up or the loss of a job, could fall within the diagnostic criteria for clinical depression. Wakefield and his colleague David Horwitz believe that for experiences such as anxiety or depression, it would be practically impossible to know if they are 'mental disorders' without investigating the context within which certain symptoms were occurring (Horwitz and Wakefield 2007).

In the absence of reliable physical tests, the diagnosis of persistent distress as a mental disorder (for instance 'depression') would seem to come down to two possible options. First, there is what could be called the 'residual category approach'. If someone has enough symptoms associated with depression, and no other plausible explanation in terms of their life events can be found, then it must be due to illness and categorised as a disorder rather than as sadness. Second, there is the proportionality approach. Here, a triggering event can be identified, such as being made redundant, but the person's symptoms are judged to be greater than would be expected and/or to last much longer than is considered normal. There are problems with both approaches. With the residual category approach, it could always be asked how thoroughly and how far back in the person's life the investigation into possible social causes was carried out. With the proportionality approach, there are value judgements to be made. Who determines what reaction to a triggering event is too big, or how long grief should last? Different societies, cultures and families will determine such judgements, which are highly relative over time and place.

If it is difficult to make a categorical decision about whether a depressed individual is suffering from a mental disorder, is it easier to identify other forms of mental distress and disturbance as distinct and pathological conditions? Richard Bentall, a professor of clinical psychology, suggests that the symptoms associated with 'psychotic disorders' are just as much a matter of degrees of variation within populations as are those of 'neurotic disorders' (Bentall 2004, 2010). Rather than symptoms being totally irrational occurrences, he views them as explainable reactions to traumatic life events. Furthermore, he questions the validity of grouping various symptoms together and presenting them as distinct illnesses such as schizophrenia, schizoaffective disorder and bipolar disorder. Instead he suggests that each symptom or experience, for instance hearing voices or feeling paranoid, needs to be attended to in its own right. Although genetic studies have shown some levels of correlation between psychotic symptoms and genetic inheritance, Bentall finds the evidence inconclusive. In addition, he points to the danger that the search for biological explanations will lead to important social factors being overlooked. Regardless of the level to which biological factors do, or do not, contribute to such disorders, this tendency to downplay the role of social factors could be an important issue.

There are many people in the population who hear voices, or who have different perceptions of reality, without attracting a psychiatric diagnosis (Beavan, Read and Cartwright 2011). Could it be that those who have supportive relationships and better coping mechanisms are less likely to need psychiatric interventions than those who don't? The work of Dutch psychiatrist Marius Romme and colleagues with groups of voice-hearers suggests that this is the case and that building trusting relationships can make a significant difference to those who are negatively affected by the experience (Romme and Escher 1993). So it could be argued that many people who are classed as having either a neurotic or psychotic condition will have much in common when it comes to the potential benefits of social support. That said, there are some differences between the experiences of those two conditions that may be significant.

Hearing voices (depending on their nature), or enjoying the energy associated with a manic high, might be experiences that an individual does not want to lose, whereas it is difficult to imagine not wanting to reduce feelings of anxiety and depression. Campaigns to recognise 'madness' as an issue of difference rather than ill-health are more likely to be supported by people with experiences viewed as psychotic rather than those regarded as neurotic. Of course, it should not be forgotten that there are also many unpleasant and frightening experiences associated with psychotic conditions.

Appropriate social support would almost always seem to be desirable whatever the diagnosis and underlying causes of mental distress or disturbance. In this chapter, it has already been suggested that social support could be related to three different aspects: distress, disorder and mental health (Payton 2009). 'Disorder' may at times be difficult to distinguish from 'distress', as, for instance, the symptoms of depression may be very similar to those of feelings of sadness and despair following a bereavement. However, the concept of disorder suggests that the disordered person might not be able to react to informal support in the same way as a distressed person; indeed the very word 'disorder' suggests uncertainty and a possible threat to personal or public safety. In this case, the feelings of friends and family could be: 'better leave it to the professionals'. But is the situation that clear-cut? People who have been diagnosed with major psychiatric disorders, whilst possibly needing crisis support from professionals, also benefit from social support, especially after a period of inpatient treatment. They don't necessarily remain 'disordered' all their lives or all of the time, and the association of mental illness with violence is much less common than the mass media might have us suppose (Walsh 2009).

From the ideas that have been discussed so far, it could be argued that distinguishing 'distress' from 'disorder' is not a straightforward matter. However, in order for people to get access to specialised help, they usually have to be recognised as having a named psychiatric disorder by a qualified practitioner. Although it might be a relief to know that one's problems can be named and treated, there is a potential downside in that this process of being labelled as psychiatrically 'disordered' can have a significant negative effect on social status and identity.

Questions of identity

Experiencing mental health problems can have a profound effect on people's identities, both as they see themselves and as they are perceived by others. Our identities do not exist in isolation, rather there is an on-going process of negotiation involving the way we identify ourselves now, the way we would like to be identified in the future and the way others actually perceive our identities. Ideally, there would be a close correspondence between all three aspects, but this is not always the case.

Consider the situation of a young university graduate working as a waitress and writing a novel in her spare time. She may identify herself as someone with creative potential waiting for the right opportunity to come along. She aspires to the identity of an intriguing intellectual who is making a significant contribution to English literature, but until she has her first book accepted by a publisher this remains largely as an ambition. At present, for the stream of tourists using the cafe where she works, she is just another waitress waiting to take their orders and that is how they treat her. Initially her friends might be willing to support her self-image as a writer doing some waitressing, but over time they may come to see her as a waitress who does some writing. How long will this young woman be able to maintain her identity as a creative writer without external validation of that identity?

Similarly, someone experiencing severe mental distress or disturbance may find their concept of their own self-identity at odds with how they are perceived by others. Unlike the young waitress, who still nurtures hope of success as a writer, they may experience a seemingly unbridgeable gap between their current devalued identity and the identity they would prefer to inhabit. The perceptions of their identity by others, especially if unfavourable, will affect the quantity and quality of their social relationships, which in turn serves to undermine their self-confidence. So there may well be a self-fulfilling aspect to the negative attitudes of others towards an individual's identity and status.

Our identities are formed, maintained, developed and changed in relation to other people and influenced by our position within social and economic structures. Thus, British sociologist Richard Jenkins (2008) approaches identity as a process of identification, something that is not fixed but is dynamic. Two key elements of this process of identification are similarity with, and difference to, other people. Friendships are largely based on perceived similarities with others (Allan 1989), whereas social distancing and rejection are based on seeing someone as 'other'. So, when considering the implications of identity for informal social support, the extent to which the person needing support, and those around them who might offer it, identify themselves as similar or different to each other could be highly significant.

American sociologists, Peter Berger and Thomas Luckman, in their classic work *The Social Construction of Reality* proposed a theory of how we gain our sense of identity and form our views of reality (Berger and Luckman 1967). These authors identified two different stages in making sense of the world and one's place within it: primary and secondary socialisation. Primary socialisation is usually influenced by parents and other close relatives and refers to the process whereby the child learns to interpret and interact with other people and the world around them as they grow up. The child's early and fundamental perceptions of reality, identity and society are socially constructed at this time by learning from and interacting with a few significant others. Secondary socialisation occurs as the individual starts to engage with the wider world. The authors in fact define this process as the internalisation of a range of 'sub-worlds'. The first significant experience of secondary socialisation is likely to be starting at school. Here, the child learns the rules of the institution and encounters other constructions of reality that may run counter to their previous experiences. However, the ideas and bonds formed during primary socialisation are usually more deeply rooted than those developed subsequently. So, for example, a child may learn to obey the teacher while at school to avoid getting into trouble, but not care particularly whether or not the teacher likes her; in contrast, at home she is very concerned to be loved by her mother and to avoid upsetting her. Similarly, at a later stage people will learn what they need to do to obtain and keep a job within an organisation, but are able to compartmentalise and separate this from other more personal aspects of their lives.

As in Jenkins' (2008) portrayal of identification as a process, Berger and Luckman (1967) suggest that each person's sense of reality and identity, although begun in their early years, is subsequently maintained and affirmed through social interactions. In the case of someone who experiences a mental health crisis, it can be argued that this process of mutual affirmation will be threatened. Experiences labelled as depression, anxiety, phobia or psychosis all imply an altered or different sense of reality. The individual may perceive the world to be much bleaker or threatening than before. They may have experiences such as hearing voices, religious-type insights or beliefs in thought-control that others cannot accept as real. Following on from this, when relatives or friends try to reassert reality as they see it, the relationship can become strained; it may even break down if the person concerned is unwilling, or unable, to accept the version of reality promoted by others. At this stage, Berger and Luckman suggest that, because they are challenging the accepted reality in a particular social context, the person becomes seen as 'deviant'. Following on from this identification of deviancy, two societal responses are possible: 'therapy' or 'nihilation'.

According to Berger and Luckman, 'therapy' is applied to the individual with the hope of changing their perceptions of reality so that they can stay within their community without threatening its world view. So 'therapy' might aim to persuade the depressed person that the world is not a dark and meaningless void, or it might try to cure the seemingly psychotic belief that it is possible to influence the material world by thought-control. The therapeutic approach requires a conceptual framework that:

- explains why individuals sometimes deviate from the accepted reality

- has an agreed means of diagnosing them as falling into this deviant category and

- offers a legitimated means of providing a 'cure' to those who have been so categorised.

If 'therapy' fails then the alternative is 'nihilation' whereby the different interpretations of reality, and those who hold them, are deemed to be 'beyond the pale'. Here, the likely way forward is to exclude or contain such people because they are incapable of changing their views. Their identity becomes that of the outsider of society or the 'lunatic' locked up in an asylum.

One possibility for people faced with 'nihilation', whether on the basis of madness, unusual religious beliefs or extreme political views, is withdrawal into a subgroup that has minimal social contact with the wider society and within which they can reinforce their own reality (Berger and Luckman 1967). An example of this is the existence of internet groups for people with eating disorders who share tips on how to lose weight and how to disguise their condition from medical professionals, which serve to reinforce the attraction of extreme weight loss (Cantó-Milà and Seebach 2011). Whilst the wider society may not like the existence of these subgroups, it may learn to live with them by incorporating explanations of their alternative world views as delusions that can be understood within an accepted frame of reference, for instance by suggesting that their beliefs arise from biological or psychological abnormalities.

The impact of identity on social support

The application of the ideas of 'therapy' and 'nihilation' to social support for mental health provides interesting possibilities for the interpretation of one person's motives to provide informal support to another (although these motives might not be recognised by those involved). If Berger and Luckman are correct, when someone we know experiences mental distress or disturbance, we would not only be concerned about their suffering but would also be unsettled by their very different sense of reality. If we are unable to change that person's perspective, we might offer informal support to help get that person into therapy. The hope being that therapy would enable them to gain a better sense of reality as we know it. Support might also be offered whilst the person is in therapy to ensure they stay with the process and to reinforce the more acceptable version of reality being offered by the therapist. After therapy, support might be offered to try to maintain the version of reality developed by the therapeutic process and to avoid the person falling back into their previous reality.

If, on the other hand, the distressed person is not able or willing to change their reality, be it hearing voices, feeling depressed or other experiences, how would the concept of 'nihilation' apply? As their reality cannot be accepted by others, it would be difficult to find a shared frame of reference, other than agreeing to differ. This is certainly a dilemma in the mental health field, where there can be a feeling that it is dangerous to 'collude' with someone's 'delusions'. As already mentioned, Berger and Luckman argue that, if the alternative reality cannot be accepted by others, it can be explained and incorporated by using the dominant theoretical framework, which could be of, amongst other things, a religious, psychological or biological nature.

Informal social support from friends and relatives becomes more problematic in this situation, as the person is seen as clinging on to an irrational, devalued and unhelpful version of reality. This is probably why some service users report that the most helpful informal support they receive is from people who have been through similar experiences to themselves and are therefore less judgemental.

Another potentially relevant aspect of identity was explored by American sociologist Talcott Parsons (1951) who developed the concept of the 'sick role'. Parsons took the view that human behaviour is constrained to function in certain ways that fit the structural needs of society. Societies generally require their citizens to be productive and seek to manage the behaviour of those who are not. When someone is clearly 'not well', other people (e.g. family, friends, colleagues, employers, doctors and welfare benefits assessors) are willing to allow that person to suspend their usual obligations and responsibilities and to support them while they are unable to function as usual. However, according to Parsons (1951), when taking on the 'sick role' the person has to fulfil certain conditions. They should view their 'illness' as an undesirable state of affairs from which they want, and have a duty, to try to recover. To this end, they should seek and collaborate with an approved form of professional help in order to facilitate a cure.

If an individual breaks their hip or suffers a heart attack they could fit quite easily into the 'sick role'; the treatment options would be fairly clear and they could expect to receive sympathy and support from those around them while they recover. In the case of someone experiencing mental distress or disturbance, such as depression or hearing voices, the situation is not so clear-cut. The first problem is that there is nothing obviously physically wrong with them, so others may find it difficult to think of them as 'ill' or 'sick'. Second, as mentioned earlier, although someone who is depressed may want to lose their symptoms, this would not be the case for everyone who hears voices or experiences the 'highs' associated with bipolar disorder, especially if they don't view them as problematic. Third, the person may not be willing to seek external help or might rather try to address their situation through alternative means such as spiritual healing, meditation or homeopathy. Some mental health problems can persist over many years and in some cases there is no 'cure', rather the person finds ways of living with their condition. For all these reasons, the sick role, as defined by Parsons, with the sympathy and support that might accompany it, may not be easily assumed by people experiencing mental health problems.

Stigma and mental distress

The work of another sociologist, Erving Goffman, is particularly relevant to understanding experiences of acceptance and rejection in social relationships. In *The Presentation of Self in Everyday Life* (1971) he considers how people manage the sense of identity they wish to present to others. In *Stigma: Notes on the Management of Spoiled Identity* (1968) Goffman looks at the processes by which certain identities are devalued and how those who are stigmatised respond to that experience. Goffman (1971) views participation in society very much like a performance in a play. There are roles to be learnt, people need to act in certain ways so that others can respond appropriately and the correct costumes and props need to be used in order to make the character seem convincing. What a person says in a particular context is only part of the performance; in order to be convincing he or she must also display the appropriate body language and attire. For some people who experience mental health problems, presenting an acceptable self in everyday life may be difficult and indeed, at times, even impossible.

One role that society offers those who do not have the attributes it values is that of the deviant or stigmatised person. According to Goffman (1968), a stigmatised identity is one that is seen as somehow less than fully human. To be stigmatised is to be marked out as unfavourably different, a person to be avoided or treated with suspicion. In the light of the earlier discussion about the process of identification being based on judgements about whom we see ourselves as similar to or different from (Jenkins 2008), stigmatised groups can be seen as extreme examples of identities that contrast with how 'normal' people would wish to be perceived. But what of those who find themselves stigmatised? Are they likely to accept the stigmatised identity or try to reject it?

Stigmatised people, suggests Goffman (1968), may respond in a number of different ways to their situation. They can attempt concealment, trying to 'pass' as normal, which involves constantly having to control and manage the information they give out about themselves. Alternatively, they may emphasise certain redeeming features such as being unusually gifted at something or being brave and determined despite their disadvantaged position. The person may internalise the stigma, feeling unworthy and insecure, which often leads to them withdrawing from social contacts and everyday activities. They might try to reduce the stigma by educating others about the reality of their situation. They may seek to overcome the embarrassment felt by others, for example by making jokes about their situation or by playing up to expectations. Another possibility is that of embracing the stigmatised identity as an alternative lifestyle or a different reality and defiantly opposing the prejudice and discrimination associated with the attitudes of mainstream society.

Recognition of the existence of stigma around mental health problems, and an understanding of the variety of ways in which a stigmatised person may respond to it, could be important in building supportive relationships. Whereas regularity and predictability underpin many of our everyday interactions, the impact of stigma can undermine these certainties. For instance, when first meeting someone known to have been diagnosed with a mental health condition, do you acknowledge and talk about this aspect of their life? If you do, how will they respond? What assumptions will they think you are making about them? To what extent do they want this to be part of their identity? Goffman's work suggests that people who are stigmatised because of mental illness can inhabit a confused status. They are advised by professionals that they could be members of society, like other people, if they are able to accept they have a problem and learn to behave in certain acceptable ways. However, they are always aware that this acceptance, if won, would be in spite of the devalued identity assigned to people like them by society, an identity that they are simultaneously advised not to deny.

Unlike certain other stigmatised groups (e.g. people born with physical or mental impairments) the person experiencing mental health problems may have spent a significant period of their life being considered 'normal' before having to adapt to their new, less favourable, status. They may not see their period of depression as anything to do with their identity and, if it is short-lived, the impact might be marginal. For those with longer-term and sometimes quite dramatic experiences of mental distress or disturbance, they may find that the reactions of others give them no choice but to occupy a stigmatised position. Whereas before their social support was part of everyday reciprocal relationships with others, it may have become a rare commodity; worse still they may encounter reactions of fear, condescension or even hostility. The fact that they have been labelled as mentally 'ill' or 'disordered' means they are at risk of being stereotyped as irrational, unpredictable and potentially dangerous, none of which is conducive to forming supportive social relationships. Members of black and ethnic minority groups with mental health problems can experience a double dose of stigma. They are particularly likely to be treated as potentially dangerous and are over-represented in compulsory admissions to psychiatric services (Browne 2009).

Becoming labelled

The foregoing discussion suggests that, if a person experiencing mental distress is finding it hard to form and maintain social relationships, this could be as much to do with their becoming labelled with a stigmatised identity as it is to do with any direct effects of their condition. And, of course, being labelled negatively and losing social relationships is not conducive to good mental health. The effect of labelling is a particular interest of American sociologist Thomas Scheff (1999), who, like Goffman, sees parallels between society's treatment of 'mentally ill' people and other stigmatised groups such as criminals. According to Scheff's analysis, social order within society is constantly being maintained and recreated by the enforcement of social norms. At an informal level, this enforcement can be as simple as smiling and nodding at someone when they are talking and behaving in an acceptable fashion or frowning at, and possibly criticising, somebody when they are not. Scheff distinguishes between behaviour that breaks certain minor social norms and behaviour that becomes labelled as 'deviant'. Some behaviours can be explained away as 'eccentric' or are not regarded as particularly serious, whereas others are perceived as so threatening or otherwise unacceptable that severe sanctions, such as loss of liberty or compulsory treatment, have to apply.

Scheff believes that much of what is considered to be 'mental illness' is behaviour that falls into a category he calls 'residual rule-breaking'. By this he means behaviours that have broken unwritten and largely subconscious norms of what is acceptable. As already mentioned, psychiatrists play an important role in dividing deviant from normal behaviour. They are socially sanctioned to make this distinction by judging whether to class individuals as 'psychiatrically disordered' on the basis of matching symptoms to diagnostic criteria. Having received a psychiatric label, the person is likely to doubt their ability to cope with future stressful situations, to be viewed unfavourably by others and, in Scheff's terms, to develop a 'career' as a mental patient. They can be seen as crossing a status line between sanity and mental illness, a line that is not equally permeable in both directions. In the case of short-term or less severe symptoms, it might be possible to recover a 'sane' status, but this can be more difficult for people who have been long-term mental hospital inpatients or who have displayed extremes of disturbed or disturbing behaviour.

The more ways there are of labelling mental conditions, and the more people sanctioned to do so, the more cases of mental illness will be recorded. So what looks like an increase in mental health problems might actually be an increase in the number of people formally labelled as disordered because there are now more services and practitioners available to diagnose and treat them. Horwitz and Wakefield (2007) contend that the large rise in antidepressant prescriptions in recent times reflects a growing trend to reclassify normal sadness as 'depression'. A similar concern has been raised by British sociologist Frank Furedi (2004), who argues that 'therapy culture' has permeated society and has undermined self- and collective determination, so that people now see themselves as weak rather than oppressed. If Furedi's analysis is correct and individuals are now more likely to view themselves as psychologically vulnerable, this would represent a challenge to C. Wright Mills' sociological mission for private troubles to be recognised as public issues (Mills 1970). For Furedi, if difficulties at work or failure to obtain decent living conditions result in depression and self-blame rather than anger and demands for political, economic and social change, then therapy can be seen as reinforcing a sense of personal vulnerability. Furedi's concerns connect with one of Scheff's ideas about health professionals performing an 'apostolic' function in which, because of the power imbalance in the relationship, they define the client's reality for them and the client accepts their version, even if it does not always fit with that person's experience.

How useful is labelling theory in exploring barriers to social support? It can help us to understand the effects of stereotyping but does Scheff's model adequately acknowledge the inner experiences of people experiencing mental distress? He admits that in seeking to establish a sociological theory of mental illness, he has ignored the individual and personal aspects of mental distress and suggests that in future a synthesis between the individual and the social aspects would be desirable. This synthesis is important for developing an understanding of social support for mental health. Conditions labelled as 'psychotic' or 'neurotic' disorders are not just about breaking informal rules of behaviour or the result of failing to meet social norms; they can be very unpleasant and disturbing experiences in their own right.

Consideration of the interaction of both individual and social aspects of mental distress seems to be necessary for understanding why social support is simultaneously necessary and yet hard to maintain during times of difficulty. If a distressed individual is having thoughts, feelings or experiences that they can't cope with on their own, this is not simply a matter of them being 'different'; rather it is a crisis situation that they want to escape from. For relatively low levels of distress or disturbance, the support offered by family and friends (if available) may be sufficient to help the person cope. In the absence of adequate social support, lower levels of distress may develop into higher levels of mental disturbance. At the more severe levels of mental distress and disturbance, it is highly likely that the person will be assessed and diagnosed as having a named psychiatric disorder by a medical or psychological practitioner. However, there is a dilemma for the person concerned. Their situation is severe enough to consider seeking professional help, but to get help at a level at or beyond primary care they will need to have a formal diagnosis, which might lead to them being unfavourably stereotyped by other people. Fear of this unfavourable labelling could lead to reluctance to seek help.

This dilemma is explored in 'modified labelling theory' (Link and Phelan 2010), which recognises that the stigma associated with being labelled as mentally ill can lead to a loss of self-esteem, a reduction in social contacts, damaged employment prospects and poorer quality of life. These difficulties can in turn make the person vulnerable to prolonged or recurring mental health problems such as depression, anxiety and paranoia. Knowing that they may encounter stigmatised responses from others, the labelled person may avoid social contact or be defensive in their dealings with other people. However, according to this theory, labelling also brings with it the benefits of being able to access various forms of therapy; it could also open up opportunities for support in addressing stressful circumstances and for gaining entitlements to welfare benefits when unable to work.

Modified labelling theory may provide one explanation for why not everyone experiencing distressing mental and emotional symptoms seeks professional help and why some people are unwilling to accept the treatment offered following diagnosis. As Link and Phelan (2010) say, it is a 'package deal' containing both benefits and disadvantages. In some cases, the reluctance to accept treatment recommendations may result in a more assertive or even coercive approach being taken by the professionals, which, ironically, whilst opening up the benefits of therapy, will also increase the stigmatic aspects of the 'package'. For social supporters there can be a tension between encouraging the individual (and others in contact with them) to think of that person as being something other than 'mentally ill' whilst at the same time accepting that they need that definition in order to receive professional support and, in many cases, to qualify for welfare benefits.

Conclusion: social understanding of mental distress

People affected by mental distress are particularly likely to experience isolation and loneliness. When forming social relationships, there is a tendency for individuals to seek out others with whom they feel they have things in common and to be wary of those who appear to be different. By separating out mental distress, mental disorder and mental health as distinct concepts, it is possible to explore different aspects of human experience. The use of the concept of 'mental disorder' has been criticised for placing certain people in a separate category rather than viewing them as part of a continuum, but without a formal diagnosis it would be difficult to access specialised professional support. Unfortunately, being classed as 'mentally disordered' does still lead to having a stigmatised identity in many sections of society, which in turn can increase the risk of becoming socially excluded and economically disadvantaged. At the level of interpersonal relationships, mental distress and disturbance could be viewed as a clash of realities between those who feel depressed or anxious, hear voices or have seemingly irrational beliefs and those who don't.

Chapter 3

Understanding social support

Introduction

Social support can appear to be largely a matter of common-sense, down-to-earth, everyday experience, so why bother with theory? When things are going well it is all too easy to take for granted the emotional and practical help provided by family, friends and others. However, as will be discussed in Chapter 7, social contacts seem to have declined in the UK over the last few decades and people affected by mental health problems are particularly likely to experience isolation and loneliness. Perhaps there are theories that can help to explain these differences and that might suggest how social support can be increased and maintained. The fields of psychiatry and psychology are informed by theories that underpin the approaches taken by practitioners; social support might similarly benefit from a consideration of some of the theories that have arisen in the field of sociology, social-psychology and other disciplines.

Distress, disorder and social support

In the previous chapter, sociological theories were presented that suggest that mental health conditions are not only a problem because of the unpleasant thoughts, emotions and experiences that can accompany them. The nature of reality experienced by the distressed or disturbed individual may not be accepted by their friends and family or by the wider society in which they live. The individual may not be able to present themselves or play a role in society in a manner that is valued by others. If their mental condition is severe enough, they may find they are cast into a stigmatised position causing others actively to avoid contact with them. Through being labelled as 'mentally disordered', the individual is associated with stereotypes of unpredictability, incompetence and even dangerousness. All of these factors can make a bad situation worse. However, the psychiatric label is also necessary and useful in obtaining specialist treatment and support. So the distressed person may simultaneously experience both positive and negative effects of receiving a psychiatric diagnosis.

The preceding discussion suggests that there are a number of issues facing an individual who is, or who could become, diagnosed as 'mentally disordered'. It is possible that social support could make a contribution at different points in the process of becoming distressed through to being officially classified as disordered. Most conditions that may attract a diagnosis of mental disorder can vary from the mild to the severe. One person might be slightly depressed or anxious and, although this spoils their enjoyment of life, they manage to keep up with everyday tasks, work and maintaining social relationships. Another person may be so severely depressed that even getting out of bed is a major effort; they may withdraw from many of the activities they formerly engaged in. Similarly, one person may hear voices or have unusual thoughts without that causing them any serious problems in their daily life, whereas another has such extreme experiences that they can no longer cope with other people or with the activities needed to sustain their existence.

The part that social support can play will vary according to the degree of distress and disturbance experienced, the qualities possessed by those offering support and the social context within which these parties operate. The relationship between social support and professional support and treatment is not always clear-cut, but is again likely to vary according to the level of mental distress and disturbance experienced and the expectations of what is appropriate within a particular society. Whereas the professional's role is fairly clearly defined in the mental health field, this is not usually the case for informal supporters. When people give freely their time and attention to support another person this might seem like a highly individual act; however there are social structures and unwritten rules that tend to influence how even something as personal as friendship is enacted.

Understanding friendship

Although some forms of social support can be organised and planned for, for instance by providing drop-in facilities and volunteer befriending schemes, the majority of social support arises in a seemingly informal and spontaneous manner from family and friends. In comparison to kinship, where it is relatively easy to define relationships in terms of the closeness of different types of relatives, it is harder to categorise friendship so precisely. This may be one reason why friendship has been studied much less than kinship by anthropologists and sociologists. Graham Allan (1989, 1996, 2008) is one of the few sociologists in the UK who has taken a major interest in exploring friendship. He acknowledges that friendship is hard to define; different people will have divergent ideas about what the term 'friend' means – some reserve it for those they know very well, others use it to describe a broad range of acquaintanceships. However, Allan argues that all informal relationships that are friendly in nature are of interest to sociologists and others who want to understand the social world. A key difference between kin and friendship relations is that the former tends to be influenced by inherited family connections, whereas the latter is voluntary in nature.

There are clearly different levels of friendship ranging from the 'best friend' to occasional acquaintance. Social support is more likely to come from those in the inner circles of emotional closeness, but sometimes a shared experience such as bereavement, or a period of depression, can bring someone from the outer circle into a closer relationship when other previously close friends may find it difficult to know how to react. In some cases there may be a deliberate effort by an agency to provide a supportive relationship, perhaps by matching the distressed person with a volunteer, which has some of the characteristics of friendship but operates within set limits. Whatever the level of relationship, an understanding of the social factors that affect patterns of friendship in everyday life can help to inform what helps or hinders social support during periods of mental distress.

Robin Dunbar, an anthropologist at the University of Oxford, has found that different species, including humans, seem to have particular limits to the size of social group they can relate to (Dunbar 2010). Dunbar's research suggests that, on average, there is an inner circle of about five people seen on a weekly basis and a further ten, less close people, who may be seen monthly. Beyond this, it is suggested that the most that can be maintained in a wider social network (including the 15 already mentioned) is about 150 people; this number includes kin as well as friends and acquaintances. Those in the outmost circle are likely to be contacted at least once a year. Each circle represents a level of intimacy and Dunbar suggests that the size of each circle is quite limited, so, if for example you already have five close friends, a newly formed close friendship is likely to displace one of the existing five into the next circle of ten and so on. The numbers of friends and acquaintances in each level of friendship, suggested by Dunbar, need to be seen as average limits to what might be possible rather than a standard that must be obtained for mental well-being.

Social network size is affected by the time available for socialising and the mental capacity needed to maintain relationships. As an anthropologist, Dunbar looked across a number of species for comparisons of social behaviour. Within the primates it is suggested that there is a significant link between a species' brain size and the size of its social groupings. It appears that humans find difficulty in maintaining and processing information about much more than 150 people at any one point in our lives. There also has to be a certain frequency of communication to maintain both strong and weak ties, otherwise relationships tend to decay. Most people have a number of demands on their time of which socialising is just one. Research on communication patterns within networks found that having a large kin network meant less frequent communication with all members and acted as a constraint on the number of friends in the person's social network (Roberts and Dunbar 2011). The same research found that contact was more frequent with emotionally close network members than those in the outer circles and that contact with emotionally close friends was more frequent than with emotionally close kin. Connections with friends require more direct contact to maintain the relationship than with kin and so are more prone to decay if attention is not paid to them.

The notion of 'decay' in social groups is very relevant to understanding the challenges of maintaining social relationships following a period of mental distress. If an individual is finding it hard to initiate or respond to social contacts, there is a danger that they will fall out of the friendship circles of former acquaintances; the longer this goes on, the harder it will be to get back in. Similarly, if family members become the main source of support, this may displace former friends, unless one party or another makes a particular effort to stay in touch.

Although social contact is valued by most people, so is time on one's own. Psychiatrist Anthony Storr (1989) writing on the role of solitude, considers sociability to be *a* hub of life but not *the* hub. There is a balance to be had between pursuing solitary activities of personal interest, taking time to rest and relax on one's own, and the affirmation and enjoyment that can be gained from the company of other people. Some people need less social contact than others, and Storr suggests that many creative thinkers and artists needed solitude in order to produce their works of genius. Despite the numbers given by Dunbar, in practice a few good friendships and some other more casual acquaintanceships may be all that many people require for well-being. The extent to which an individual is either introverted or extroverted in nature is likely to play a part in the size of social network and the frequency of contact that suits their needs. However, if an individual starts out with very few friendships, any loss of relationships resulting from a period of mental distress could lead to a significant decline in the social support available to them.

Social structures and friendship

Friendship and interpersonal relationships are affected by, and central to, social structures. Social structures consist of both institutions and established ways of doing things, which, as mentioned earlier, tend to become accepted as a socially constructed reality through processes of socialisation. Institutions range from large-scale, such as government departments, schools, hospitals, organised religion and commercial organisations, to small-scale, including families, local associations, shops, workplaces and health centres. Social structures as 'ways of doing things' can be seen in Goffman's (1971) descriptions of the norms and expected behaviours encountered in everyday life and in special situations. So, for example, there are unwritten 'rules of engagement' when you happen to meet a neighbour in the street, such as the expectation that the conversation will start off on some fairly safe topic such as the weather. When visiting a GP there will also be expected modes of interaction that will make the encounter feel appropriate and safe and are likely to emphasise the professional role of the GP. Similarly, Parsons' (1951) 'sick role' describes an expected way of behaving when health issues limit the ability to function as normal. Allan (2011) suggests that these social structures contribute to the nature of the 'immediate social environment', which shapes and constrains the experiences of the individual who occupies it. So although friendship may seem to be a matter of personal choice, that choice is made within the context of the social environment.

Social structures are the component parts of society and society is rarely static. As economic and industrial development has taken place, societies have changed and increasingly the forces bringing about that change are viewed as global in nature. Sociologists, social historians and many lay people have come to view the 'modern' world as a place in which social life has become more impersonal, fragmented and individualistic than in former times (Giddens 1990; Allan 2008). Studies, particularly of Western society, have pointed to the decline of traditional communities and a move from living in extended families towards nuclear family units, or indeed to increasing numbers of people living alone (Office for National Statistics 2011). Local shops, pubs and other facilities have declined as out-of-town shopping centres have blossomed. People are less likely to work near to home or to know their neighbours than in the past. At the same time, the home, with its technological resources of household appliances, televisions and computers, has become the focal point of many people's lives (Chaney 2002).

What is the impact on social life of this ever-changing environment that shapes and constrains the formation of social relationships? Allan (2001) agrees with other commentators that the nature of the social world has changed, for instance with geographical proximity being less of a requirement for friendship, but believes that friendship is as important as ever, despite the apparent individualisation of personal life. In fact, with there being less structured certainties in life, such as a secure job and lasting family relationships, Allan suggests that people are constantly having to redefine their identities and that friends play an important role in that process. However, as a person's life situation changes, the relationships associated with that former life may diminish or cease, while new ones more in line with the person's changed identity and status may develop. It could be argued that if our society is now more fluid in terms of geographical and social mobility than in former times, there are more possibilities for mental health service users to 'reinvent' themselves rather than being typecast and stigmatised within their community of origin.

Drawing on my own experience of growing up in a small market town, it seemed to become widely known through local gossip who, at some point in their lives, had been patients of one of the three mental hospitals that served the area. This then became a major feature of how some townsfolk viewed these people. Subsequently, upon moving to the nearby city and working in a mental health service, I noticed that a number of people from my hometown, and from similar surrounding small towns and villages, who had spent some time in a mental hospital were now living in the poorer section of the city. On the one hand, this represented a reduction in the quality of their lives; the physical environment was noisier, dirtier and generally less aesthetically pleasing and rates of crime were higher. On the other hand, in the more anonymous and culturally diverse inner-city they were not so clearly marked out as different, and many were accessing day centres or similar facilities; some seemed to be developing friendships with other service users in contrast to being isolated in their previous neighbourhoods.

The above personal example endorses the notion that many service users experience 'social drift' (Rogers and Pilgrim 2005), meaning that after experiencing mental health problems they could be judged to have gone down the socioeconomic scale. As income drops, they are more likely to be living in rented accommodation in the less fashionable districts of inner cities, their employment prospects are diminished and they are less able to partake in the social and cultural activities they previously enjoyed. So, in terms of social and economic status, service users have suffered. However, by finding common ground with other service users and by removing themselves from the constraints of their communities of origin, at least some may be able to enjoy a better social life. Again drawing on my own experience of working in a community mental health setting, I was struck by how many friendships developed between service users with very different social class backgrounds, based on the common experiences of using the mental health system.

The social drift of service users into deprived inner-city areas and down the social scale raises important issues of social inclusion and exclusion. The fact that social drift occurs suggests that a number of service users are experiencing social and economic discrimination, which, in combination with any direct effects of their mental distress, has disrupted their previous life-course and has led to a form of 'ghettoisation'. This was recognised by the Labour government in power in the UK in 2004, which launched a major report into social exclusion and mental health (Social Exclusion Unit 2004). This report took a broad view of service users' experiences, encompassing not only use of health and social care services, but also the impact of family, community, employment, finance and housing. The report's recommendations included actions that would increase participation in all aspects of life so that broader social networks could be built and maintained. Although the report acknowledged the support that service users gave to each other, its emphasis was on participation in 'mainstream' activities and it was not clear whether it valued the role of on-going peer support. In fact, one part of the report refers to some service users being 'restricted' by 'only' having contact with fellow users.

Helen Spandler (2009) warns against the social inclusion agenda being used to dictate how service users should lead their lives. Although it is clearly right to seek to overcome social exclusion, there are dangers in government officials and others with positions of power laying down the law about what it means to be socially included. Spandler points out a number of issues associated with the concept of social inclusion. There is an implicit belief that being in the 'mainstream' is predominantly unproblematic and desirable; people with mental health problems should want to be included. There is also an implication that there is an agreed form of the mainstream society with common goals that satisfy the majority of people. Inclusion is viewed as fundamentally good for mental health and this is seen to apply to all who are currently excluded. These assumptions can divert attention from the conflicts in society that may cause distress, instead shifting the focus to how individuals can be integrated within it.

The vision of society presented by social inclusion is rather one sided and simplistic; there are other perspectives. If, for instance, Karl Marx's (1971, first published 1844) analysis is considered, a whole new vista opens up. Here, rather than being a harmonious whole, society is portrayed as the site of bitter divisions where there are huge inequalities in wealth and power, with exploitation of the many by the privileged few, and in which alienation is the natural state of being. Whether or not a Marxist analysis is adopted, research points to the conclusion that the more unequal the society, the higher the levels of distress experienced by its population (Wilkinson and Pickett 2009). So rather than inclusion being seen as a universal good, the question needs to be asked: what sort of society are people being encouraged to sign up to?

There is a danger that, in the name of social inclusion, there can be an unhelpful focus on the individual correcting their deficits rather than examining the negative impact of the damaging structures of society (Spandler 2009). Those currently excluded who do not cooperate in an approved manner may be seen as dysfunctional. Although choice might be identified as the important issue, some choices may be seen as more worthwhile than others. There can also be a coercive element; the policy issues around reducing welfare benefits and increasing expectations of seeking employment are especially contentious in this respect. By contrast, an approach that combats social exclusion allows more attention to be paid to the barriers that prevent service users leading lives that give them satisfaction, making a valued contribution and maintaining a sense of meaning. There are many parallels here with social models of disability, which aim to make society less disabling rather than identifying individuals as needing to be 'fixed' (Beresford 2009). Issues of social inclusion and exclusion are revisited in Chapter 7.

Social networks and social capital

If society can be seen as containing a number of social networks, some complementary to each other and some competing, then the goal of inclusion or integration within an idealised and homogenised notion of society seems too simplistic. Instead, there would be a need to identify social networks that the service user would benefit from joining. Social networks can be as small as a group of friends or as a large as national or international associations of people who share common interests. People who are excluded from informal and formal social networks that would be of value to them could be said to be denied access to 'social capital'.

The concept of social capital (Bourdieu 1986; Putnam 2000) is a shorthand way of referring to the advantages that can be derived from being connected with other people. It is a somewhat 'messy' concept in that it is used in different ways and has been added to by successive writers (Webber 2005). The personal connections associated with social capital tend, like friendship, to involve a sense of mutual trust and expectations of reciprocity. There can be collective advantages, such as being able to band together to bring about some form of change or to resist an unwelcome development. There are also individual advantages such as tip-offs about jobs or housing becoming available or inside knowledge about how to be successful in gaining employment or promotion within a company, as well as information about services, products and leisure opportunities likely to be of personal interest. So access to social capital can be seen as empowering on many levels. Of course, social capital can operate in ways that are detrimental to service users, the most obvious example being NIMBY (not in my back yard) campaigns to prevent mental health facilities being developed in 'desirable' residential areas.

Robert Putnam (2000) identified two different forms of social capital: bonding and bridging. Bonding social capital refers to associations of like-minded people with similar backgrounds or concerns. Bridging social capital refers to situations where a diverse range of people are brought together through some form of shared interest or common cause. The concerns in the *Mental Health and Social Exclusion* report (Social Exclusion Unit 2004) about mental health service users having most of their social contact with other service users can be seen as wanting to encourage a move from bonding to bridging capital. Support from fellow service users can be very helpful, as they are likely to be empathetic and to have useful knowledge of dealing with mental health issues. However, developing contacts and associations beyond the world of fellow service users opens up connections with other social networks that may be useful in terms of making choices about employment, housing and leisure activities.

Some of the links between social networks, social capital and mental health will be explored further in Chapter 7.

Social support and health outcomes

Although social support theories suggest the benefits of being connected with others, and many people will have an intuitive feeling that being supported by friends and relatives must be good for mental well-being, is there any evidence to back this up? A range of studies show that being part of a socially supportive network is not only good for mental health but that there are physical health benefits too. There is evidence of the negative effects of loneliness, which can lead to depression, anxiety, decline in cognitive ability and problems with dealing with stress (Cacioppo *et al.* 2010). Neurological studies suggest that the 'social pain' of isolation is experienced in the same neural pathways that transmit the feeling of pain from physical injuries (Eisenberger *et al.* 2006). Feelings of loneliness are associated with raised blood pressure and higher levels of harmful cholesterol in the blood (Hawkley and Cacioppo 2010). Lonely people are likely to suffer from a lack of adequate sleep and to have problems adhering to medical guidance and treatment (Segrin and Passalacqua 2010). So loneliness not only makes people unhappy but also increases their risk of physical illness and early death. At the time of writing, there has been media interest in a study (Cacioppo and Cacioppo 2014) reporting that feelings of loneliness carry twice the risk factor for mortality compared with obesity, making it a condition that should be a major public health concern on a par with campaigns for weight loss and smoking cessation.

By contrast to the effects of loneliness, social support has a positive effect on physical and mental health. The concept of social capital has been used to explore the links between social connectedness and health. In some studies, social capital has been measured in terms of an individual's feelings of trust in others and their perceptions of the availability of support and reciprocity; other studies have looked at the numbers of people within a person's network and their engagement with civic activities (Murayama, Fujiwara and Kawachi 2012). Reviews of a range of studies seem to suggest that it is the former personal appraisal of social capital that is most strongly linked with positive mental health outcomes, especially in reducing the incidence of anxiety and depression (Bassett and Moore 2013; De Silva *et al.* 2005). However, this is not to say that civic engagement and having dense social networks are irrelevant, as it is often through these means that people meet others with whom they can form trusting and reciprocal relationships. For women in particular, it seems important to their mental well-being to have social contacts outside of the family, possibly because for them the family is particularly associated with having caring responsibilities (Cable *et al.* 2013). A large-scale USA study over a ten-year period found that individuals who started out with the lowest amount of social support were twice as likely to become depressed than those who started out with high-quality relationships (Teo, Choi and Valenstein 2013). Similarly in the UK, people who reported a lack of someone to talk things over with were more than twice as likely to have high scores on measures of anxiety and depression compared with those who had supportive relationships (Harrison *et al.* 1999). The recovery of people diagnosed as having schizophrenia is also positively influenced by social support (Harvey *et al.* 2007). The positive effects of social support for both mental and physical health are such that help with developing social relationships is increasingly being recommended as a health intervention (Bassett and Moore 2013; Economic and Social Research Council 2013).

Enabling social support

The discussion so far makes social support sound somewhat instrumental with an emphasis on reciprocity, maintaining a shared sense of reality, defending shared interests and improving personal health and well-being. Does this undervalue the quality of human relations by ignoring emotional issues of empathy, concern, liking and loving? Do people only look out for 'their own' or can they have sympathy for outsiders? People who are employed in caring services such as nursing and social care are paid to undertake 'emotional labour', but what do theories have to say about the conditions under which people are likely to offer social support voluntarily?

Close friends and family are an obvious source of support, but sometimes the person experiencing mental distress does not want friendships or family relationships transformed into a 'caring' role (Henderson 2001); in some cases friends and relatives may not have the ability to offer appropriate support. So in addition to, or instead of, using professional help, the distressed individual may seek informal support from outside of their immediate social circle. Sometimes that support is needed from others in the community, a workplace or an educational institution, so that the individual is able to continue with or resume activities that are important to them. In those settings, the potential helpers may not have a close relationship with the person needing help but for various reasons find themselves in a supportive role.

The literature on supportive relationships suggests that there are differences between the expectations of support offered within close friendships and that provided by acquaintances and others who are less emotionally involved. Anthropologist Joan Silk (2003) distinguishes between exchange relationships and communal relationships. Exchange relationships assume some direct reciprocity ('tit for tat') in the short term and are typical of relationships that are not emotionally close. In contrast, communal relationships are associated with close friendships and would be devalued by the expectation of immediate reciprocity or 'payback' (Silk 2003). Social support for people with mental health and other serious problems seems to rely, at least to some extent, on altruistic behaviour. At those times when one party is distressed or confused and in need of help, the relationship cannot always be an equal one. Therefore, unpaid support relies on the helper being prepared to give time and energy without expectation of any return, other than possibly the satisfaction of knowing that he or she has been of help to others.

Philosophers have been concerned with questions of human nature, individual motivation and choice for many centuries. One of those questions concerns whether an individual ever chooses to act out of anything other than self-interest. It can be argued that even seemingly charitable acts are carried out to make the givers feel better about themselves. Immanuel Kant (1959, first published 1785) believed that the only selfless acts are those carried out through a sense of duty and that if the person is motivated by feelings of compassion they are not being selfless because they are acting to meet their own emotional needs, such as feeling useful.

The theoretical construct of altruism offers an explanation as to why at least some people are prepared to provide support without thought of personal gain. Whereas some philosophers such as Kant have argued that true altruism is hard to find, on a practical level it does seem useful to attempt to understand the circumstances under which actions that at least appear to be altruistic take place. Evolutionary theories suggest that kinsfolk may be motivated to provide mutual support because of a shared interest in preserving a common gene pool, but this doesn't explain why non-relatives are prepared to offer support to others. C. Daniel Batson (2010) conducted a range of psychological experiments designed to explore the motivation for empathetic feelings and altruistic helping behaviour. He concluded that this motivation is derived from emotions and cognitive awareness associated with parental nurturance. The desire to nurture offspring becomes generalised to others who are seen as having support needs. In contrast to theories that suggest that people are motivated to help others similar to themselves, Batson believes that the key motivational factor is the recognition of characteristics and needs in others that are similar to those of the helper's actual or potential offspring. This recognition then triggers feelings of concern and empathy that can lead to supportive behaviour.

Other writers also challenge the view that human nature is intrinsically egocentric and selfish. Economist Kaushik Basu (2010) sees cooperative behaviour as the norm in human societies. Contrary to extreme free-market ideas that unfettered individualism provides the best route to economic prosperity and stability, he posits that the opposite is the case; trust and cooperation are essential for successful economic and social development. However, Basu warns that altruism can be a force for both good and evil; members within one community can behave altruistically, for instance sacrificing themselves for their peers in order to oppress or overwhelm members of another community.

American writer Alfie Kohn (1990) also argues that altruism and empathy are a basic part of human nature and that aggression and fierce competitiveness are not inevitably dominant in all human societies. Kohn reviewed a number of social-psychological experiments concerning altruism and concluded that altruistic behaviour arose from a combination of certain environmental and personal factors. People are less likely to offer help if they believe that there are others who could do so, or if they are in an anonymous setting such as a city as opposed to a small town. In the immediate situation of someone needing help, personal exposure to that person's needs, or a direct appeal on their behalf, is more powerful than hearing about them indirectly. The clearer it is that the person is unhappy, the more likely it is that they will be offered help. Personal aspects of the potential helper that are likely to promote altruistic behaviour include: positive mood, confidence in their own ability and guilt about a recent personal action. There are also particular personality characteristics that seem to favour altruism amongst helpers in the longer term, the main ones being: self-esteem, a reasonable level of assertiveness and good interpersonal skills (Kohn 1990).

Conclusion: understanding social support

Social relationships exist at many levels, ranging from a small, intimate inner circle of friends and family to a much larger and more impersonal outer circle of acquaintances. Whereas close relatives or friends offering support may act out of a sense of love or duty, others may do so because of the combination of their personal traits and characteristics with features of the social context within which help is required. If the factors that encourage people to act altruistically can be understood, this may provide some useful pointers for enabling social support. The nature of modern society challenges the formation and maintenance of social relationships but makes them as important as ever, especially for people whose lives have been disrupted by mental health issues.

Chapter 4

Close up and personal

The importance of supportive relationships

Introduction

Contact with friends, neighbours, colleagues and family can be very important for mental well-being, but at times of emotional crisis and on-going disruption of everyday life it can be difficult for those concerned to know how to act for the best. If someone experiences prolonged mental distress, the nature of their relationships with family members, friends and others is likely to change; their bonds may be either strengthened or weakened by the need for support and it is likely that there will be a rebalancing of relationships. In some cases, a relative or a friend will take on the role of 'carer'. However, other, and sometimes less close, relationships may also play a role in maintaining well-being. This chapter builds on the previous discussion of social support for mental health, with a particular emphasis on the role of personal relationships. This focus has been chosen because close, confiding relationships are important to both reducing the risk of experiencing mental health problems and promoting recovery from them. Although largely focused on the role of friends and family, many of the ideas presented in this chapter are also applicable to the relationships found between colleagues in the workplace or between students and staff in educational settings.

In this and the subsequent chapters, in addition to drawing on published research and other works relevant to social support, the content has been informed by my own experiences of working in a community mental health setting, as well as those gained from teaching and researching on mental health issues over many years. To illustrate some of the points made I will draw on two pieces of personal research: a three-year, qualitative study of the support given to students with mental health issues (Leach 2004) and a nationwide survey on attitudes to mental health support conducted in collaboration with The Open University colleagues (2011) following the broadcast of two television programmes on mental health issues developed in partnership with the BBC.

It should be emphasised that, in contrast to large-scale randomised control trials for evaluating the effectiveness of pharmaceutical and some psychological treatments, most of the research on social support is small-scale and qualitative in nature. Given the huge variation in needs, experiences, personalities and social contexts between different individuals, it is not appropriate, or even possible, to come up with a general prescription for the most appropriate and supportive social relationships. However, this chapter will explore some of the issues that can aid understanding when mental distress or disturbance affects a person's life and it is hoped that this will be useful in helping social supporters to reflect on the situations in which they may find themselves.

Informal support from family and friends

In a survey about support for mental health problems in the UK (The Open University 2011) 71 per cent of 376 respondents reported receiving informal support from family and friends; their comments show that this support was very important to them, especially in terms of having someone with whom to talk things through and for receiving practical assistance:

> 'Quite often talking is the best form of therapy and having someone who knows you, who you can confide in and can talk back to you on a personal level based on the fact they know you, can sometimes be very comforting.'

> 'I could not survive without the day-to-day support of my neighbours and friends. They help my daily functioning and control my money and medication.'
>
> *(Respondents, The Open University survey 2011)*

Earlier studies (Faulkner and Layzell 2000; Milne 1999; Harris *et al.* 1999) have also indicated the importance of informal social support in meeting a number of areas of need. This support seems to fall within five broad categories: engaging in friendship, providing emotional support, constructing meaning, offering practical advice and giving material assistance.

Friendship

Friendship, or companionship, as a type of social support refers to individuals spending time together or staying in contact largely for the pleasure of each other's company. It should be noted that friendship could also be viewed as the basis on which other social support is built (Barnes and Duck 1994); people are more likely to turn to someone they know and trust in a crisis than a stranger. However, it is possible to offer advice or practical support to someone without being their 'friend', as in the case of people who undertake voluntary work. It is also possible to conceive of personal relationships that don't involve significant emotional support or the giving of practical assistance, but that still feel as if they are 'friendships'; for instance two men who regularly go to football matches together but who never discuss personal issues. So it does seem worth considering friendship as one aspect of social support, even though it will often overlap with others.

As well as being pleasurable in itself, friendship also seems to be helpful in providing some form of distraction when the time is right, which can help people break out of cycles of depressed or anxious thoughts:

> 'My friends who were there to talk, to make me cups of tea, to share their experiences or just take my mind off things with a silly movie and lots of cake!'
>
> *(Respondent, The Open University survey 2011)*

Too much time alone can lead people to being overly introspective and concerned about relatively minor matters that may then get blown up out of proportion. Loneliness, especially when experienced over long periods of time, has many detrimental effects on physical and mental health and has been associated with depression, anxiety, feelings of stress, anger, paranoia, pessimism and lowered self-esteem (Hawkley and Cacioppo 2010). Loneliness is not just a matter of how few people are known, it is also dependent on the strength or weakness of the relationships that do exist. Enjoying the company of other people seems to meet a basic social need and is part of what respondents to a research project on recovery from mental health problems described as 'being good to yourself' (Borg and Davidson 2008). In order to preserve this quality of friendship, there seems to be a need for reciprocity in relationships, 'give and take', which may be difficult to maintain if friends or partners become too much like 'carers' (Henderson 2001):

> 'I have close and caring friends but I try not to use them for support too much because I don't want them to feel like carers rather than friends. I have used them in life-and-death situations when I need someone I trust to take control, but this is rare.'
>
> *(Respondent, The Open University survey 2011)*

Graham Allan (2001) points to the key role of friendship in affirming a person's identity; friendships are often chosen and nurtured because they help each party to maintain a similar world view and to reinforce their self-images. Friendships also seem to develop between people with a similar economic and social status and therefore hierarchies tend to be avoided in close relationships. It may be due to this tendency for friendships to be formed and maintained on the basis of equality of status that some mental health service users report changes in their friendship networks:

> 'Some friends and family were very supportive, but without fully understanding the problem I was having. Some friends were less than welcoming to me... Since being involved with services and meeting like-minded people, I have made a number of new friends who have been an enormous support and have been able to empathise with me.'
>
> *(Respondent, The Open University survey 2011)*

As illustrated in the above quote, companionship and friendship can lead to emotional support. A number of research studies have pointed to the importance of close, confiding relationships for good mental health and this seems to apply whether or not the person has a recognised mental disorder (Harris *et al.* 1999; Harrison *et al.* 1999; Singleton *et al.* 2001).

Emotional support

Emotional support, as part of informal social support, consists largely of listening, showing empathy and concern and perhaps trying to lift the person's mood. Faulkner and Layzell's (2001) user-led research on coping strategies described acceptance by others as a key component of the emotional support needed. They felt that this could also act as a stepping stone to self-acceptance by the recipient. When acceptance by others was accompanied by a sense that they also had insight into the person's situation, this was seen as particularly effective. Such understanding might come from personal experience of mental health issues or through taking the time to learn about them. Contact with others who have shared similar experiences and who can then empathise with them is certainly valued by some service users:

> 'Where would I be without my wonderful friends that I have since made through illness.'

> 'Sharing my experiences with other service users helped me realise I was not alone in the way I felt. I also wasn't judged or isolated.'
>
> *(Respondents, The Open University survey 2011)*

Communication specialist Brant Burleson (1994) has suggested that the provision of comforting messages within a relationship serves to maintain an individual's self-esteem and positive mood in the face of daily struggles, stresses and disappointments, all of which, according to some researchers (Hutchinson and Williams 2007; McIntosh, Gillanders and Rodgers 2010; Tessner, Mittal and Walker 2011), can have a negative impact on mental health and exacerbate a range of mental health problems. Burleson has analysed the content and impact of a range of comforting messages and describes them as being on a continuum from 'sophisticated' to 'non-sophisticated'. Sophisticated comforting messages are the most effective, as they are focused on the recipient's needs and show sympathy and understanding of their situation. By contrast, non-sophisticated messages are largely focused on the giver's perspective on the situation and influenced by their need to provide interpretations and to dispense advice. The level of sophistication in comforting messages also affects how supporters feel after an interaction, both about themselves and the recipient of their support, with those giving less sophisticated messages tending to feel less satisfied and more critical of the recipient (Burleson 1994).

In social interactions, some people can become quite skilled in opening up emotional issues for discussion, but is it always good to talk? An excessive focus on emotional problems may be unhelpful. Conversations that mainly focus on past problems may not be beneficial, as they can encourage rumination on the negative factors in a person's life, which may increase their levels of depression (McIntosh *et al.* 2010). Another danger of focusing on emotional issues, highlighted in research by Derek Milne (1990), is that other people may unhelpfully make the person's situation seem more catastrophic than it actually is. They may overemphasise the impact of a stressful factor and imply that the person will not be able to cope without professional support, thus undermining their confidence in using personal coping strategies. In the end, deciding how far to go in exploring difficult feelings is probably a matter of degree, as not acknowledging the other person's emotional state would not be experienced as empathetic behaviour and could be as damaging as making it seem too important.

The role of emotions within the family is an especially difficult facet of social support. One aspect, expressed emotion, has received particular attention, especially in relation to the chances of recovery after being treated for schizophrenia. However, expressed emotion has also been identified as significant for coping with other diagnosed psychiatric conditions such as depression and eating disorders. Patients returning to families with high levels of expressed emotion, often largely critical in nature, have been found to be at greater risk of relapse and hospital readmission than those whose families had a lower level of emotional expression (Buzlaff and Hooley 1998). This has led to the development of family education interventions by health professionals in order to bring about changes in the emotional dynamics between the service user and their family (Carr 2006):

> 'When I first became ill my mother was very angry. She has since made enormous changes in her behaviour and continues to try… which has been a great help to me.'
>
> *(Respondent, The Open University survey 2011)*

If, as mentioned earlier, the recipient is comforted by 'sophisticated' communication of reassuring messages that acknowledge their own experiences and views (Burleson 1994), this raises the question of what happens (as may have been the case of the mother in the quote above) when the potential supporter does not perceive the mentally distressed person's views of their own reality as legitimate. The idea that personal relationships are based on maintaining a shared reality was mentioned in Chapter 2; it was also suggested that if this broke down the responses could be those of either 'therapy' or 'nihilation' (Berger and Luckman 1967). 'Therapy' here refers to attempts to bring the individual back into the accepted or mainstream reality, whereas 'nihilation' involves denying the legitimacy of the different views, reality and identity held by a person who 'fails' to take up or respond to therapy. The sociological use of the term 'therapy' in this context, although it embraces psychological treatments, also covers a wide range of formal and informal social control measures intended to counter the 'deviant' perspectives of the distressed or disturbed person.

The use of sociological terms such as therapy, nihilation, deviant and social control, can give an impression of an Orwellian system of authoritarian repression. In practice, these processes can be operating within the context of close circles of families and friends who are genuinely concerned and upset about members who are depressed, anxious or experiencing psychotic symptoms. Ironically, the studies of expressed emotion suggest that showing you care too much about how someone has changed might be more harmful than taking a somewhat more relaxed but supportive attitude to the situation (Bentall 2010).

Meaning

The previous section of this chapter has already touched on issues of shared and divergent realities following the experience of mental health problems. After having experiences that challenge their former ways of experiencing and interacting with the world around them, service users can feel a strong need to construct meaning in their lives. Although this is a personal journey, it takes place within a social context:

> '…sharing experiences to help me understand what I was going through, and how to make sense of it. This support was largely from my mother, brother and particularly my sister-in-law who was studying occupational therapy at the time.'
>
> *(Respondent, The Open University survey 2011)*

In Chapter 2 the social construction of meaning and reality was described as taking place in two separate processes: primary and secondary socialisation (Berger and Luckman 1967). Primary socialisation starts from birth and sets the individual up with their basic perceptions of the world and how to interact with it. Secondary socialisation occurs as the person encounters, and needs to engage with, contexts beyond the immediate family such as school, college, workplace and community. Subsequent mental health issues may alter the perceptions derived from these earlier processes; the world may seem a darker, more threatening environment than before and the individual may doubt their abilities to move towards goals of their own choosing.

Social support can play a role in a form of re-socialisation during which old meanings are recovered or new ones discovered. Faulkner and Layzell's (2000) research respondents described the finding of meaning as gaining a sense of belonging, which could be in relation to a group of friends, family or to a service such as a drop-in centre or other facility. For these respondents, part of this sense of belonging was the feeling of caring about others and knowing that they, in turn, were cared about. This yet again reflects the importance of reciprocity and equality in maintaining on-going relationships. It would seem that friendship and family relationships can play a key part in supporting the individual's identity by helping them realise that they are not alone in their experiences and struggles:

> 'Knowing that people actually cared and were concerned. Also I found out that other family members had been through depression and more people than I ever would have realised have been there too. It is more common in society than people will admit, due to the attached stigma and labelling.'
>
> *(Respondent, The Open University survey 2011)*

So, although there can be an intense and disturbing personal journey through mental distress, the meaning of that experience and its impact on an individual's identity are likely to be affected by the reactions of, and relationships with, other people. Although some people have embraced the status of 'service user' or 'survivor' of the psychiatric system and have become active in attempting to change it (Campbell 2009), others have emphasised the importance of having a 'normal life' rather than being defined by their mental health problems (Borg and Davidson 2008). Whatever the pathway chosen, other people will have a role to play in supporting the recovery of meaning in an individual's life.

'Recovery' is a term that has seen increasing usage in the world of mental health over the last 25 years or so. Starting with the experiences of service users such as Patricia Deegan (1988) in the USA, the concept of recovery has more recently been incorporated into national and regional mental health policies, statements of service aims and professional literature on mental health. In contrast to less optimistic approaches, which seek merely to reduce symptoms and minimise the risk of harm, recovery has represented a positive outlook on the prospects for leading a meaningful and enjoyable life following a period of mental ill-health. However, there is a danger that, in such widespread adoption, the term becomes one that is applied too indiscriminately, attracting mere lip service rather than actually making a difference to people's lives (Craig 2008).

As someone who had received a diagnosis of schizophrenia, Patricia Deegan (1988) found herself comparing experiences with Brad, a man who had quadriplegia following an accident in which he broke his neck. Both were classed as disabled in respect of their conditions, but they also shared a feeling that it should be possible to regain a sense of self and purpose despite their situation. Deegan describes recovery as an active personal process, not something that is 'done to' individuals. However, she believes that it is possible to identify some of the factors that provide a nurturing environment within which any sparks of hope can be kindled. Although she was addressing her remarks to rehabilitation settings, her suggestions also have relevance to the role that family and friends can play in the process.

First, it needs to be recognised that recovery will often be in the form of small steps forward and that there will also be steps backward; this is not failure but the reality of trying to move on. Despite setbacks the door should be kept open, offering the chance to pick up at the point where the person left off, so as to try again and again. Second, each person's journey will be different; although they can learn from the experience of others, they need the freedom to make their own pathway to recovery. Third, other people with experience of mental health problems or disability who are a few steps ahead in their recovery can be important sources of hope to those who are struggling with their own journey. Finally, Deegan (1988) suggests that the attitudes of others are very important and that it is helpful to avoid divisions between 'normal' and 'abnormal', rather acknowledging that everybody has their vulnerabilities that they need to try to overcome:

> 'Colleagues supported my difficulties in remembering or comprehending what was required of me. They were grateful for anything I was able to achieve and encouraged me when I stumbled.'
>
> *(Respondent, The Open University survey 2011)*

By helping to give meaning to distressing experiences, and through encouraging hope that things can get better, it would seem that informal support can play a useful role in recovery.

Offering advice

The giving of advice is an interesting area of social support as it is almost always a well-intended action but is also one that carries a number of risks:

> 'Other people who have not experienced the full extent of a mental health problem can think that it is just like when they are feeling down, so they may not offer appropriate support or advice.'
>
> *(Student respondent, Leach 2004)*

Offers of advice and practical assistance are the most concrete expressions of being helpful. Ironically, such offers may thus be unwelcome for some recipients, as the experience can reinforce feelings of dependency and inadequacy, particularly in individualistic cultures that place high value on achievement through personal effort. Many people seem to be comforted by knowing that support is available to them but are less happy about being the actual recipients of support (Bolger and Amarel 2007). As mentioned earlier, 'less-sophisticated' support messages that pay little attention to the needs and feelings of the recipient but are strongly related to the needs of the giver to put their view across are likely to leave both parties feeling dissatisfied with each other (Burleson 1994). So giving advice is something to be approached with caution unless that advice has been sought; even then, how that advice is given should be carefully considered:

> 'People have talked to me. I can't be sure they listened. Lots of advice.'
>
> *(Respondent, The Open University survey 2011)*

There are a number of reasons to be wary of giving advice as an informal social supporter. The advice given may not be applicable to the person's situation because they don't have the same experiences, resources or outlook on life as the giver of that advice. The advice given may be biased by the giver's beliefs rather than being based on a rational appraisal of the recipient's needs and their situation. Also it may conflict with the advice given by others, for instance: 'you don't need medication' or alternatively 'you need medication'; 'you need help' or 'you just need to pull yourself together'. Giving advice may meet the helper's needs to try and fix the situation but not the needs of the person being 'helped'. Giving advice may convey a sense of impatience and a simplistic understanding of the situation, thus sending out the message 'you ought to be better by now' without actually enabling the person to find what they need in order to recover. There is also the danger that constantly giving advice may undermine the person's decision-making abilities and reinforce their feelings of helplessness and dependency (Seligman 1990).

Nevertheless, when someone close to us is distressed or seemingly lost in confusion we naturally want to help and to give them the benefit of our experience. Also, a flat refusal to provide advice when asked might be unhelpful when trying to build or maintain a supportive relationship. It is useful here to recognise the difference between giving informative advice and interpretative advice. Informative advice can be along the lines of giving information about where and how to get welfare benefits, how to access medical and social services or where to find drop-in facilities such as voluntary sector run day centres. Interpretative advice is likely to consist of telling people how they should be feeling or what is causing their problems or to be solution-focused in suggesting what they should be doing, for example: 'don't dwell on your problems' or 'try to get out more'. The latter type of advice is likely to be more problematic in that it assumes that what worked for the giver will work for the receiver:

'It is difficult to know who will have empathy – my experience is that most people just don't understand that my anxiety might be deeper than theirs.'

(Respondent, The Open University survey 2011)

Of course, even informative advice can be used selectively in a biased manner, for instance, by only providing information on one category of support services, be they medical, psychological or social in nature.

Any interaction between two people has certain underlying dynamics, and this applies to giving advice as much as to other types of behaviour. Writing from the psychological perspective of transactional analysis, Eric Berne (1964) suggested that communication between two people can be analysed as transactions between their different internal ego states of parent, adult or child. The parent ego state can be nurturing, controlling, critical and authoritative. The child state can be playful, fearful, angry, rebellious, helpless and irresponsible. The adult ego state is, by contrast, more rational, evaluative and open to negotiation. Regardless of the actual age or relationship status of each party, they may relate to each other in all the possible combinations of different ego states: child to child, adult to adult, parent to parent, parent to child, parent to adult, child to adult. Significantly, Berne says that the ego state of one person can trigger a corresponding one in the other. So, for example, if the helper stays in 'parent mode' and dispenses authoritative advice to the distressed individual, this may reinforce that person's 'child' ego state rather than helping them to access their 'inner adult'. This would suggest that, if giving interpretative or solution-focused advice, it might be best approached along the lines of 'this is how I see it – what do you think?'

Giving material assistance

Some service users have placed high value on receiving practical material assistance for many aspects of daily life such as: shopping, cooking, cleaning, help with childcare, getting out of bed, being lent money and being accompanied to appointments (The Open University 2011; Faulkner and Layzell 2000). In some cases, the amount of assistance given amounts to some people performing substantial roles as a 'carers'; one person described the considerable range of informal help that she had received:

> 'Someone to talk to, staying with me to keep me safe, encouraging me to eat, helping me get to appointments, listening to me, understanding me, encouraging me to carry out daily living tasks like showering, getting dressed.'
>
> *(Respondent, The Open University survey 2011)*

For others, material assistance will just consist of occasional help with tasks that they would otherwise find difficult or impossible on their own. If an individual is not meeting their basic needs for income, food, secure housing, personal hygiene, etc., this not only increases their feelings of worthlessness, it also imposes a practical impediment to meeting their higher level needs such as for sociability and personal development (Maslow 1970). Borg and Davidson's (2008) research with a small set of service users identified an approach of 'just doing it' and 'making life easier' as part of the recovery process. The same research emphasised the importance of leading an everyday 'ordinary life' away from clinical settings; practical assistance can clearly play a role in making this possible.

How practical support is given seems to be quite important to the recipient:

> '[I received support from] …family and some friends although their lack of understanding of mental health and their ignorance/fear at first was a problem.'
>
> *(Respondent, The Open University survey 2011)*

Some of Faulkner and Layzell's (2000) respondents described feeling uneasy when practical support was given to them without the giver conveying any sense of empathy for what they were going through. This is supported by another piece of research on patients receiving treatment for low back pain (Semmer *et al.* 2008) where the emotional meaning of giving and receiving practical assistance was found to be very important. Practical support that was carried out in a manner that made the recipient feel cared about, showing empathy, respect and acceptance, was highly valued for its emotional significance. This suggests that, despite breaking social support down into different component parts for the purposes of analysis, the experience of receiving that support is a holistic one and that all the components mentioned in this chapter are interconnected.

As mentioned earlier in relation to giving advice, being the recipient of visible support can make some people quite uncomfortable (Bolger and Amarel 2007). This would seem to be related to the recipient's self-image and their current situation; some people are quite open about their need for support whereas others see it as a sign of personal weakness and they hate to feel that they are pitied by others. As in other aspects of friendship, it would seem that reciprocity is important.

Friendships survive by maintaining a balance in the amount of practical help being exchanged over the long term, although in the short to medium term friends may be prepared to help out during difficult periods without expecting any direct reciprocation. In contrast, there seems to be less concern about reciprocity when help is given by family members (Allan 1996).

Giving and receiving social support

So far this chapter has focused on the nature of social support, but under what circumstances is that support either sought or avoided? Whatever may have caused a mental health problem in the first place, the social context within which the person is situated can have a significant impact on their well-being. The fear and stigma attached to mental health problems can act as a disincentive to sharing thoughts and feelings, even with close relations and friends, because of the anticipated negative impact on those relationships. One service user responding to a question about using support from friends or family commented that he did this:

> '…not as much as I should because I am ashamed of my inability to get better and hide it. People talk to me and offer help where they can, but I'd hate to bother them and besides, I'm not sure there's much they can do.'
>
> *(Respondent, The Open University survey 2011)*

Similarly, a university student stated that:

> 'It is much easier to talk to a stranger than to sit down and talk about certain personal issues with someone who knows you. Part of your self-respect is to promote a healthy picture of yourself to friends, not to show all the eyesores that only you can see on the inside.'
>
> *(Student respondent, Leach 2004)*

There is wide variation in the extent to which different people will be open with others about their problems and needs; some may seem almost too ready to share their troubles with anyone they encounter, whereas others want to keep their problems from even their closest friends and family. In between these extremes it is likely that many people are selective about what personal issues they discuss with the various people they know.

American sociologists Brea Perry and Bernice Pescosolido (2010) undertook detailed quantitative research on who gets approached within social networks to discuss mental health issues as opposed to other important matters. This research was based on a sample of 171 individuals with diagnosed mental health conditions such as: schizophrenia, schizoaffective disorder, bipolar disorder, major depression, general adjustment disorder, generalised anxiety disorder and dysthymia. The results showed that, on average and regardless of diagnosis, each individual discussed either health or other important matters with three other people, and that health matters in particular were only discussed with one or two people. Family members (used by 42% of respondents) were more likely to be thought of as being important in health discussions than health professionals (24%) or friends (19%).

The links between having close health discussants and the individual's views on using mental health services and their feelings of optimism about personal mental health and recovery were explored in the same research project. If the individual had a close relationship with the other person with whom health issues were discussed, he or she was more likely to be satisfied with the services they used, to report an increase in their levels of mental health and to be more optimistic about their chances of recovery. A difference emerged between respondents who had diagnoses of severe and psychotic conditions and those with less severe conditions. The former were more likely to place trust in medical practitioners if they had close health discussants, whereas for the latter no significant effect was found. Respondents with psychotic conditions tended to restrict discussion of health issues to family members, and this may be because they encountered stigma when talking to other people about their problems. However, associates who had been through similar mental health issues were valued as health discussants (Perry and Pescosolido 2010).

The study conducted by Perry and Pescosolido (2010) suggests that having social networks that only involved discussion of 'important matters' did not have an impact on positive views about treatment, mental health and recovery, whereas those that included discussion of health issues did. If these findings can be applied to people experiencing mental health issues in other countries, such as the UK, it would seem that discussing health issues with a friend or relative is an important element in promoting recovery.

Is social support a type of informal psychotherapy?

Social support offers a lot of things that are not available in a psychotherapeutic relationship, but if, as research suggests, certain people are sought out for discussion of mental health and emotional issues then how similar are these discussions to what might occur in a therapy session?

> 'What this student wanted was to be listened to by someone who really cared about her, not the kind of relationship you get in a counselling situation.'
>
> *(Student respondent, Leach 2004)*

The quote above suggests that the speaker did not believe that a psychotherapist or counsellor could convey the genuine empathy that could be shown by a friend or relation. While it is true that the boundaried nature of the client–practitioner relationship sets limits on emotional involvement, empathy is considered to be an important quality of therapists' work (Palmer 2000). It is likely that support given by someone who is paid to do so is perceived differently to support that is offered voluntarily, even though the paid therapist often does feel empathy for their client. On the other hand, the fact that the person is seeing a professional may give the latter's interpretation of their situation a certain weight.

In a supportive encounter, whether it is with a therapist, friend or volunteer, time will be spent in establishing the helping relationship, even though one context will be formal and the other informal. Unlike social support, the whole context of a therapy session is formal and task-oriented with a specific period of time set aside and, quite often, an agreed number of sessions offered. The therapy session will take place in a room set aside for the purpose rather than in the individual's home or another informal setting such as a cafe. It is more likely that there will be an agreed set of tasks and goals during the period of therapy than would be the case for informal support.

Looking beyond the context within which interactions occur, the talk-based aspects of social support provided by friends and family members have both similarities to and differences from the types of support that are provided by counsellors and other psychotherapeutic practitioners (Barker and Pistrang 2002). In both cases, the parties need to establish, or develop further, a helping relationship based on empathy, trust and mutual respect. Similarly, there is likely to be a shared concern to make sense of, or give meaning to, the distressed individual's experiences. In psychotherapy, the helper will draw on a body of theoretical knowledge and associated practical techniques to discover this meaning, whereas the informal supporter is more likely to attempt this by using knowledge derived from their own life experiences and observations. Both approaches may attempt to go beyond discovering meaning to try to enable changes that will overcome, or at least reduce, the individual's distress and vulnerability. In the therapy relationship, change may be encouraged by the therapist who guides their client to develop insights into what is holding them back and how they can overcome these obstacles. As has already been suggested earlier in this chapter, informal supporters are more likely to offer advice and guidance in order to try to bring about such change (Barker and Pistrang 2002; Milne 1999).

Unlike mental health practitioners, who are trained to set clear boundaries with their clients, it is much less likely that friends, relatives and other informal supporters will enter a helping relationship with clearly defined limits in place. So what level of involvement is appropriate for social supporters engaged in the process of finding meaning and promoting change? My own research found examples of concerns about the dangers of well-meaning people dabbling in 'amateur psychotherapy' and this is something that many professionals are likely to be worried about. One university-based counsellor spoke of:

'...tutors or others who are inappropriately trying to do too much, perhaps using limited counselling skills... Without awareness, staff can develop false dependency relationships with students, or in good faith set up relationships with students whose needs they can never fulfil. This situation can be serious when they get out of their depth and there is a crisis, the relationship breaks down and they demand and expect immediate help for the student from the Counselling Service.'

(Counsellor, Leach 2004)

Informal social support is not subject to the scrutiny, regulation and requirements for training and accreditation that apply to psychotherapy;

that is both its strength and its weakness. It means that the support is readily available in natural environments, but that the quality of that support can be highly variable.

Some insights into the processes involved can be gained by looking at the issues that arise when volunteers provide befriending support, as this is a situation when boundaries and expectations tend to be made explicit and it is often arranged to make up for a lack of existing social contact. A UK study interviewed befrienders and befriendees in order to explore the nature of the befriending relationship (Mitchell and Pistrang 2011). Some of the findings have implications for what might be helpful in other social support situations. Responses showed that it was considered important for the befriender to show empathy, but not for them to enter too completely into being empathetic; having a sense of perspective was seen as healthy for the relationship. Befrienders sometimes had to make an effort to be non-judgemental, but both parties recognised how important this was in making the relationship feel safe. The relationship was not entirely like a natural friendship in that the befriender might avoid disclosing personal information and did not expect the support to be reciprocal. When the befrienders felt that they were in the role of 'carer' the relationships tended to feel less like a friendship, as they were particularly aware that the focus was on the other person's needs, not their own.

The same research found that, in common with some forms of psychotherapy, befriendees valued the opportunity to talk about thoughts and feelings quite freely, providing a sense of release and enabling greater clarity. Befrienders could play a valuable role in asking questions and encouraging the befriendee to weigh up various options, but not in a directive manner. Another way in which the befriending relationship resembled a psychotherapeutic one was that it was established with the knowledge that it would be time-limited and that, at some point, both parties would need to work towards its ending (Mitchell and Pistrang 2011). Although this aspect would not be mirrored in relationships with friends and relatives, there could be lessons to be learnt. For instance, it could apply when both parties want to move back to a more reciprocal relationship after a period of crisis during which the relationship has become more one of carer and cared-for. In this instance, instead of working towards the end of the relationship, the goal could be to achieve a rebalancing and perhaps a broadening of the scope of their relationship.

Supporting change

One of the aims of social support, in common with psychotherapy, can be to bring about change for the distressed person. However, there are challenges in any situation where one party feels they need to help another by encouraging them to face up to difficult truths and supporting them to change the way they think, feel and behave. Psychotherapist John Heron (1990) has outlined six types of intervention that he sees as the main approaches that may be used in such situations by therapists and other types of supporter. Although each has its own distinctive features, Heron sees them as being used in conjunction with each other during a therapy session or a similar period of interaction. Some may seem (and probably are) more appropriate than others for use by informal supporters. Building on the previous discussion of the nature of social support, it is possible to use Heron's six categories to review different types of interventions that can occur in informal support interactions:

Prescriptive interventions attempt to direct the behaviour of the individual and as such may feel unwelcome unless that person feels they wish to relinquish control to another. However, there are certain situations, particularly when the behaviour in question poses a risk of harm to self or others, in which it would be impractical to be anything other than prescriptive. Ideally this would be a short-term solution to keep the person safe until a point when they can become more self-directed; being subject to prescriptive interventions over a sustained period of time tends to lead to angry rebellion or 'learned helplessness' (Seligman 1990). In the earlier discussion on giving advice (which can be a form of prescriptive intervention) it was noted that advice that came from the giver's perspective without much consideration of that of the recipient tends to have a damaging effect on the relationship.

Informative interventions underpin much of what seems to be valued within social relationships, as they aim to develop the distressed person's knowledge and understanding of their situation and to help them find a sense of meaning. As previously mentioned, the role of friends and relations who are able to draw on their own experiences of dealing with distress and mental health problems seems to be particularly helpful. As in the case of a prescriptive intervention, there is still a power imbalance in that one party is presumed to have knowledge or insight that the other either does not possess or is not able to access during a period of crisis. Nevertheless, the transfer of that knowledge or insight can help the more vulnerable person become increasingly resourceful and self-directed. As Heron (1990) points out, there is a balance to be had between being too informative or not informative enough.

Confronting interventions are perhaps the most challenging and contentious of the six types covered by this framework. As described by Heron, this is not an aggressive confrontation but rather a deliberate attempt to raise someone's awareness of aspects of their behaviour or thought processes that are seen to be holding them back. Although the intention behind the intervention may be well meant, the very fact that the person was not aware of the issues raised prior to their revelation is likely to result in them experiencing some level of shock. The expectation that this may be the case can lead the supporter to feel anxious about giving this type of feedback. This anxiety may lead them to either 'pussyfoot' around the issue, which will confuse the recipient, or to 'clobber' the person concerned with comments that seem over-critical (Heron 1990). This is a very real issue for those close to someone experiencing mental distress or disturbance who have to decide whether or not to raise an issue and, if so, how best to do it.

Cathartic interventions might also need to be approached with caution by social supporters. Here, the intention is to enable the person to discharge painful emotion. Strong emotions are not easy to deal with and friends or relations, unlike professional therapists, are unlikely to have supervision and support sessions to help them debrief and deal with their own feelings arising from the interaction. There is a danger that rather than a 'clean' discharge of emotion, the person may experience a 'messy' re-stimulation of former distress, thus holding them back rather than enabling progress. Some personal relationships do enable catharsis to occur but this is not something to artificially engineer into a social support situation. Those therapists who do use this technique have the benefit of professional training and support, which should equip them not only to open up painful emotions, but also to do so in ways that feel safe and can be brought to a satisfactory conclusion within the session.

Catalytic interventions, in contrast to the two preceding types, are likely to appeal to many social supporters, as these are focused on promoting self-discovery, self-directed living, learning and problem solving for the distressed person. However, it should be noted that, in contrast to therapy sessions, which are usually carefully constructed to enable these processes, social interactions are more likely to consist of a high proportion of advice-giving and expression of opinions (Milne 1999). To overcome this it would be necessary to ask open-ended questions and to encourage reflection on current and past experiences as well as exploring future possibilities (Heron 1990). This is the sort of interaction that Burleson (1994) refers to as 'sophisticated' communication; it is based on listening to what the recipient of support is saying and working with it in a non-judgemental manner.

Supportive interventions, the last of Heron's categories, are at the heart of social support relationships as they are aimed at affirming the worth and value of the individual, appreciating their qualities, attitudes and actions. Indeed it could be argued that such interventions may have greater value coming from social supporters than therapists, as they are initiated by people who are not paid to offer support but do so because of connections of kinship, friendship or voluntary work. However, as Heron points out, messages about an individual's worth and positive qualities may be difficult for them to hear or believe, especially when they are feeling depressed. To some extent, it may be helpful to ensure that such messages are quite specific and can be backed up with examples, rather than being generalised and vague (Heron 1990).

Although each of Heron's six supportive interventions has been presented from the perspective of the social supporter helping the distressed person to change, they could equally well be seen as means by which the distressed person attempts to bring about changes in the way that other people relate to them. For example, they could inform family, friends or colleagues of patterns in their behaviour that are adversely affecting the individual's health or are holding back his or her recovery. They could equally focus on supporting changes in attitudes and behaviour in others that are more beneficial to the well-being of the individual.

In everyday social situations, it would feel unnatural to use these interventions deliberately as a therapist might. However, each represents examples of behaviour that are found in interactions between people in the home, at work, in educational settings and in recreational situations. Awareness of these can be helpful in developing a more proactive approach to social support rather than relying on instinctive responses that are not always helpful.

Relationships, caring and mental health

In this chapter, much of the focus has been on the support that might be given by those people who are in a close personal relationship with a distressed or disturbed individual. These relationships are extremely important but can be challenged by the experience of mental health problems and there can be significant emotional demands on the person providing support. A considerable overlap can exist between being a supporter and being a 'carer' and the former role can shift into the latter at times of crisis. The role of carer is required when someone is no longer able to look after themselves (Larkin 2012) and is often undertaken by close relatives. However, as previous examples quoted by service users in this book have shown, friends and neighbours can also take on aspects of the caring role.

Much of what has been written in health and social care literature about the caring role relates to the experiences of caring for people who are ageing or who have long-term physical impairments and conditions that deteriorate over time, such as multiple sclerosis and dementia. By contrast, many conditions labelled as mental health problems can fluctuate across the lifecycle and individuals can experience varying degrees of recovery from them. Supporting someone who experiences severe mental distress can pose different challenges to those raised when an individual requires help with their physical needs. Traditionally, the role of carer has been associated with providing support for basic needs such as washing, dressing, toileting and feeding. In caring for someone with a mental health problem, it is relatively rare (although not unheard of) to have to meet such needs; the support is often more emotional and social in its nature (Pirkis *et al.* 2010). However, it is not uncommon for developing physical conditions to be accompanied by mental health issues such as depression (Barnard and Lloyd 2012), or for mental health and physical health problems to co-exist, and that situation seems to have a particularly draining effect on carers (Hastrup, Van Den Berg and Gyrd-Hansen 2011; Pakenham 2011).

The UK, in common with most other countries, has moved away from long-term, inpatient mental health care to a model of care in the community backed up by community support teams and crisis beds for acute episodes. Community care relies on a mixture of professional and informal care, which, in a number of cases, has replaced levels of support that would have formerly been provided within a hospital setting. As the input of health and social care professionals is generally quite time-limited, much of the 'care' element inevitably falls on family and friends. The National Health Service and Community Care Act 1990 gave formal recognition to the role of carer and subsequent UK legislation required that carers' needs be assessed, although it did not follow through with making the resources available to meet these needs (Glasby 2007).

A UK government policy paper *Recognised, Valued and Supported* (Department of Health 2010) encouraged those with responsibilities to identify themselves as carers in order to have the value of their contribution and their needs recognised. However, different people will vary in the extent to which they wish to identify themselves as 'carers' and this policy paper recognised that one factor is the stigma attached to mental health problems. Another factor, not mentioned in the paper, is that formalising the role of carer can put a close relationship on a different footing to one based on a more informal and impromptu approach that exists in friendship or the intimate one that exists in marriage and partnerships (Henderson 2001).

The impact on the carer can vary greatly and, despite ideas of 'carer burden' in the literature on the topic, not everyone undertaking the role will view it as burdensome (Hastrup *et al.* 2011). Nevertheless, there can be emotional and practical costs to the carer and resulting difficulties for the person being supported. If caring over long periods of time, carers can experience isolation, reduced income and diminished job and pension prospects. There is also concern about children who find themselves becoming carers for a parent and who, as a result, miss the opportunities available for their own social and personal development (Department of Health 2010).

Apart from the impact on carers, those receiving informal care face challenges in their relationships. Service users report social contacts, including those with relatives, to have both beneficial and harmful effects (Green *et al.* 2002). For instance, partners are not always sympathetic during periods of distress and this can result in distancing and dismissive behaviour (Alexander 2001). Placing responsibility onto the distressed individual for their problems often leads to making critical comments, can have a negative impact on the relationship and diminishes the chances of recovery (Grice *et al.* 2009; Kuipers, Onwumere and Bebbington 2010). One person's response to the question 'what else might have helped' in The Open University (2011) survey was:

> 'Probably a local approachable group for family and friends. If family and friends were not so frustrated with me and noticed my mood was getting worse rather than holding stigma that I was "putting it on" or "being lazy".'
>
> *(Respondent, The Open University survey 2011)*

The above respondent clearly felt that he or she was held back by the attitudes and behaviour of precisely those in close contact who might be expected to be the most supportive in times of trouble. Elizabeth Kuipers and colleagues from the UK's Royal College of Psychiatrists (Kuipers *et al.* 2010) suggest that how family members and other informal carers appraise the situation can have a significant impact on the mental well-being of the service user. They propose three types of relationships that typify different modes of informal caregiving in mental health: positive, emotionally over-involved and critical/hostile.

Positive relationships between carer and service user tend to have been on a good footing before the mental health problem became manifest. The service user is still viewed first and foremost as a person rather than being defined by their problems, which are seen as being unusual for, rather than typical of, that person. The carer is able to offer support whilst still feeling and showing respect for the recipient. Positive carers can ask others for support for themselves and are likely to retain at least some of their existing external interests. Although these carers can feel stressed by the situation they are in, they do have useful coping strategies and are less likely to become clinically depressed.

Emotionally over-involved relationships can arise through the carer's feelings of loss, shame and guilt and they are likely to blame themselves (at least to some extent) for the service user's problems. Parents, even of adult offspring, are particularly at risk of becoming emotionally over-involved and over-protective as carers if their sons and daughters develop mental health problems. Such carers tend to focus negatively on what has been lost and they are likely to give up their other interests in order to provide a high level of protective care. They are less likely to ask for support and thus may lose their own support networks; they run the risk of becoming isolated and depressed.

The third of Kuiper *et al.*'s categories is that of *critical and hostile relationships* between carer and service user. This relates to the problems of expressed emotion in families linked to higher relapse rates that have been mentioned previously, which, as some other authors (McFarlane and Cook 2007) have suggested, could more accurately be described as 'expressed exasperation'. In critical relationships there is likely to be a background of a poor mutual relationship prior to the mental health crisis. Any problematic behaviour tends to be seen as typical of the person rather than unusual, meaning that help may not be sought until things have become too difficult to cope with. This tendency to delay can be added to if carers adopt an 'avoidant' coping strategy, such as doing nothing and waiting in the hope that things will improve by themselves. The carer is likely to blame the person with mental health problems rather than themselves for the situation and to view themselves as relatively powerless to effect any change. The pressure is on the person to get better through his or her own efforts. Given the degree of criticism involved, the distressed individual is less likely to approach the 'carer' for help or to confide in them. Carers falling into this category can experience low self-esteem, anger, resentment and depression (Kuipers *et al.* 2010).

Being a carer for someone with mental health problems does present significant personal challenges and it is important that the carer looks after their own mental health and is looked after by others. As the previous discussion has indicated, there are a number of factors influencing how well the caring relationship works out. In any stressful situation there seem to be three important factors affecting how that stress is managed: the nature and severity of the situation or event itself, the person's appraisal of that situation and the effectiveness of the coping strategies that they adopt (Lazarus 1999). Different people will have differing degrees of tolerance to stress, but most will reach a point where it can feel overwhelming if they don't know their limits and don't feel able to ask for external support.

When social support is not enough

A key question for individuals providing social and family carer support for someone who is becoming increasingly distressed or disturbed is when to seek professional help. This is effectively saying 'we have reached the point where neither you nor we can cope alone with what you are going through'; it is not a step that people take lightly. If triggered too readily, it can risk making a minor setback seem like a catastrophe and might unnecessarily medicalise problems arising from daily life. On the other hand, if left too late, the person's situation may have deteriorated much further than would have been the case if help had been sought sooner. In a Canadian study, Addington *et al.* (2002) found that attempts to seek help in the early stages of psychosis tended to be unsuccessful and it was only when full-blown psychotic symptoms became manifest that help was obtained; this was then through emergency admission to a psychiatric facility, which is often a traumatic experience for all concerned. The same study found that only half of the sample of 86 families with a member experiencing psychosis sought help before the psychotic symptoms became more dramatic. They argue for better education of the public and general health practitioners about the early signs of psychosis. This would allow for early intervention rather than having to treat the condition when the person's mental and social functioning had been significantly impaired.

O'Callaghan *et al.* (2010) found that family members were closely involved in ensuring access to treatment but also found significant delays between initial symptoms and eventually seeking and receiving professional help. Models of stress, appraisal and coping (Lazarus 1999; Lazarus and Folkman 1984) may help to explain why not all mental health problems are presented to professionals, and why those that are may have been lived with for some time before external support is sought.

First, decisions about seeking professional help are linked to the nature of the problem itself. When a family member is slightly depressed, anxious, obsessive or is having strange thoughts, but is not causing significant difficulties to others and is able to function as normal much of the time, then help may seem unnecessary. If the effects are more dramatic with temper outbursts, actual or threatened violence or self-harm, severe social and psychological withdrawal and a general breakdown in everyday functioning, then help is likely to be sought with some urgency.

A second factor is the appraisal of the situation made by the distressed person and by their close relatives or friends. As mentioned earlier, if problematic behaviour is seen as typical of the person concerned, it may not be viewed as symptomatic of an underlying mental health issue (Kuipers *et al.* 2010). Similarly, if someone is depressed following bereavement, redundancy or other forms of loss, this could be appraised as a normal reaction to life events and not something that should attract a psychiatric diagnosis. However, if, as discussed in Chapter 2, the person's distress goes on for longer or is more extreme than other people judge to be reasonable, it might be interpreted as an illness. Research on the beliefs about mental health problems held by members of the general population indicates that, not surprisingly, when people define the problems as symptoms of an illness they are more likely to seek help for themselves or others (Rüsch, Evans-Lacko and Thornicroft 2012; Henshaw and Freedman-Doan 2009). Severe depression and the types of disorder classed as 'psychotic' are most likely to be viewed as illnesses, in contrast to stress, grief and drug addiction, which are not (Rüsch *et al.* 2012).

In addition to the intellectual appraisal of the nature of the problem and its meaning, there is also the question of how people feel about it. Lazarus (1999) points out that there is an emotional element to the appraisal of any situation and suggests that this should not be dismissed as an 'irrational' reaction, as emotions tend to flow from a person's evaluation of events. Whether relatives feel guilt, anger, blame, sorrow, pessimism or optimism in relation to the distressed person will shape how they react to them and what decisions they make about involving health professionals or other external sources of support.

Family members will have different styles of coping, some of which are more successful than others. Avoidant coping is not a very useful strategy; hoping that the problem will go away if it is ignored tends not to work in cases of mental distress (Kuipers *et al.* 2010). Emotional coping may help the relative to get by and can be an important element in managing a difficult situation, but may not be sufficient in itself. Practical coping consists of getting the information, skills and support resources in place to help address the situation that is the source of the stress. Experience of successful coping in the past will boost the person's confidence that they can cope in the present or future (Lazarus 1999).

The factors linked to appraisal and coping interact to influence help-seeking decisions. The same level of challenge in a situation will be appraised differently by different people; their interpretations of it and feelings about it, combined with the nature and strengths of their coping mechanisms, will influence whether and when they will seek external support. However, external factors can also affect their appraisal of their situation and will determine the extent to which they have to cope on their own. The messages that are conveyed by health professionals, whether in person or through guidance in advice leaflets, websites and mental health awareness campaigns are likely to affect attitudes to seeking help. Typically, people do not want to bother busy health practitioners with problems that they fear will be seen as too trivial. Family members may worry that they will be judged as causing or contributing to their relative's mental health problem (Lefley 1996). They may also be afraid that contact with health services may lead to the person concerned being stigmatised as 'mentally ill' and possibly to being treated in a locked ward (the influence of films such as *One Flew Over the Cuckoo's Nest* on public perceptions of mental health treatment should not be underestimated):

> 'One or two clients fear that it is the first rung to involvement with psychiatry or to admitting to being psychiatrically ill. When needing a second opinion I have found that it is less upsetting for the student to say "I think you should see our medical consultant who is a psychiatrist", rather than "I think you should see our psychiatrist."'
>
> *(Counsellor, Leach 2004)*

Despite these concerns, friends and relatives often do decide to persuade an individual to seek professional help or even to contact services themselves on that person's behalf (with or without their permission or knowledge). A number of respondents to The Open University survey (2011) indicated that it was someone else who initiated their contact with the mental health system. Respondents to this survey were asked what advice they would give to someone facing a mental health crisis. One key message was to avoid thinking that use of professional support should mean withdrawing from other sources of support. As one service user advises:

'Get professional help, but confide in people closest to you also. It's hard to get by with no support from your friends or family, the medical profession can't hug you and make it better.'

(Respondent, The Open University survey 2011)

The first time that someone is seriously affected by a mental health problem is likely to be difficult on a number of levels including: getting the problem recognised, gaining access to suitable treatment or support and working out the relationships between service user, family and professionals. Carers can find themselves in an ambivalent relationship with healthcare professionals. The concept of community care relies on their involvement and yet a number of carers report being marginalised by professionals and finding it difficult to obtain support when a crisis situation develops (Askey *et al.* 2009). Here the sharing of confidential information is a big issue and practitioners may feel uncomfortable about receiving information about their patient from family members. They are also likely to have ethical concerns about passing information about the patient on to their family.

Confidentiality concerns are important if the service user is to feel they can trust the mental health practitioners who are treating them. The fact that professional support can take place in a confidential setting means that the service user has a safety valve for their feelings away from the family:

'Mum…offers emotional support but I try not to use her because I'm afraid of being a burden. I'm honest with the professionals I see and tell them what is going on in my head and self-harm issues. It's too traumatic for family.'

(Respondent, The Open University survey 2011)

Some attempts have been made by service providers to clarify what information can be shared with family members and the circumstances under which this takes place, but research findings indicate that the situation is not clear-cut. There is a recognised role for a named relative when someone is compulsorily admitted to hospital under the powers given in mental health legislation, and family members or friends can be identified in care plans when a patient is discharged back into the community. Some service users favour the use of advance directives in which they specify how they would like to be cared for in times of crisis. Muhlbauer's (2002) research on the family's role during a mental health crisis suggests that there can be a move from confusion, fear and uncertainty in the early stages to growing awareness, confidence and ability to find useful strategies as time goes by. Unfortunately, the combination of limited resources and uncertainty about confidentiality and patients' rights poses difficulties in developing means by which mental health professionals can aid the family's growth in this way. Despite the reported problems of informal carers and professionals working together, social support would seem to be an essential element in any context where social exclusion and isolation may result from the experience of mental health issues (Green *et al.* 2002).

Conclusion: involving family and friends

In this chapter, the nature of social support from family and friends has been explored in some detail and five key components were identified: friendship, emotional support, meaning, advice and material assistance. Health issues only seem to be discussed with one or two people, but those discussions appear to be important in getting the most out of support services and in promoting recovery from mental health problems. Although some aspects of social support could be seen as covering the same ground as aspects of psychotherapy, there are also significant differences between the two, which it is important to acknowledge and maintain. A particularly intense form of social support arises when one person becomes the 'carer' for another. The caring relationship is one that places demands on the carer, but also can be rewarding, particularly if the carer can find the right appraisal and coping mechanisms to deal with the stress involved. Carers and social supporters need to know their limits in terms of what situations they should be dealing with on their own and what they personally can cope with. When these limits are reached it is important that supporters can draw on and work alongside external sources of help. Despite the focus of this chapter being largely on family and friends, much of what has been said has relevance to the supportive relationships that can develop in educational and work settings and these are the topics of the next two chapters.

Chapter 5

Education matters

Support in schools, colleges and universities

Introduction

Engagement with education offers exciting opportunities to learn new things, to develop and mature as a person, to meet like-minded people and generally to acquire the skills, knowledge and attributes that will improve an individual's chances of having a good life. Inevitably, some aspects of each person's potential will be measured and labelled according to their achievement of qualifications. Thus, time spent in education can lead to experiences of inspiration, excitement, pressure, stress, exuberance and disappointment; as the title of this chapter states – education matters! Whilst in education, students are subject to the same challenges in life as other people, plus the demands of learning new things and being assessed through coursework and exams. If these challenges are not coped with, they can have a negative impact on a student's academic achievement. In turn, academic failure can have a negative impact on the individual's future life, including feelings of low self-esteem and the likelihood of diminished career prospects. If social support can play a role in supporting educational achievement and personal development, it could then also have a positive impact on present and future mental well-being. As the main focus of this book is adult mental health, most attention is paid in this chapter to further and higher education. However, as experiences at school can influence later life, we start with a brief consideration of mental health and social support within schools.

Education and mental health

Population surveys tell us that levels of mental distress vary across the life-course. Around 10 per cent of children aged 5–16 in England and Scotland have been reported to have a diagnosable mental disorder (Green *et al.* 2005). In adulthood, the numbers experiencing mental health problems increase. A large-scale population study in England shows a rise in probable 'common mental disorders' towards middle age (largely experiences of anxiety and depression, not all of which will be recorded as requiring a medical diagnosis). In the 16–24 age group, 17.5 per cent of those surveyed reported symptoms of common mental disorders in the previous week. There is a peak in the 45–54 age group, with 19.9 per cent reporting symptoms; after this things tend to improve so that only 10.6 per cent of the 65–74 age group were affected. The reported levels of probable 'psychotic disorders' (such as schizophrenia and bipolar disorder) are much lower than those for 'neurotic disorders'; in the 16–24 age group, 0.2 per cent have reported psychotic symptoms in the past year and the levels of incidence reach a peak of 0.9 per cent in the 35–44 age group (McManus *et al.* 2009). Interestingly, a previous large-scale survey of England's adult population reported that adults who had achieved a qualification level of two A-levels or above were twice as likely to report psychotic symptoms compared with the general population (Meltzer *et al.* 1995). This suggests that such symptoms could be more commonly encountered amongst university students than their peers of a similar age who are less qualified.

Although health professionals tend to be wary of giving young children a psychiatric diagnosis, there is no doubt that mental disturbance and emotional distress can be an issue. Within any school there will be a significant number of pupils experiencing mental distress. Whilst some try to cope on their own or with support from family, others are referred to a school counsellor, their GP or children's and adolescents' mental health services because of the serious nature of their distress or disturbance (Green *et al.* 2005). The nature of the problems encountered tends to vary according to the age group but can include anxiety, disordered conduct, low mood and eating disorders (Gelder *et al.* 2005). Problems at home can lead to both mental distress and difficulties with what would be considered a normal pattern of childhood development. Problems at school, especially with bullying, can also have a very negative impact on well-being. As problems that begin in childhood can affect the process of maturation and persist into adult life, there have been a number of schemes in the UK aimed at providing support to children and their parents at increasingly earlier stages of development. Many of these, such as the 'Sure Start' scheme and 'Children's Centres', can be seen as a form of social support (although formal rather than informal in nature), as they offer advice, guidance and support to parents in group settings in the community (Bagley 2011).

Social support in schools

Although school children with the more extreme and dramatically presented problems are likely to be referred to specialist agencies for support, there will be many more who are affected by mental health issues in a less obvious way and who may not access help from any type of health professional. In one study, in the south west of England, 45 per cent of the adolescents surveyed said they would consider seeking help from a teacher or other school professional if they were feeling down and 97 per cent felt they might approach them if they were worried about use of alcohol or drugs (Farrand, Parker and Lee 2007). By comparison, 55 per cent said they might approach a health professional about prolonged low mood, but only 3 per cent would consider taking alcohol or drug concerns to that source of support. Of the various potential sources of support within the schools, the pupils' form tutors were identified as the most likely to be approached for help.

As teachers are seen as a significant source of support, it follows that they need appropriate knowledge and skills that go beyond academic instruction. The quality of the teacher–pupil relationship is very important, with personal warmth and supportiveness improving pupils' engagement with school and promoting emotional well-being and academic achievement (Cooper 2011a). The way that teachers communicate with pupils is significant, but so too is the physical layout of the classroom and the encouragement of peer support within the class. Specific techniques of behavioural management may be needed for pupils who display challenging behaviours, but developing a general approach to teaching that supports emotional and mental well-being can make a significant difference for a wider range of pupils. Conversely, teachers who develop poor relationships with pupils tend to exacerbate behavioural and emotional difficulties in the classroom (Cooper 2011a).

Some children with mental health issues will be designated as having special educational needs and may be supported in the classroom by teaching assistants, learning support assistants or other special needs staff. This demonstrates a way of attempting to integrate children with special needs within mainstream education. However, as with any social or other type of support that is quite visible to others, it does mark the recipient out as different and could lead to stigma and isolation. The staff offering this support have much in common with many other social supporters. They do not always need to have a specific qualification to undertake the role and can feel disadvantaged in the hierarchical structure of the organisation where staff with professional qualifications and roles have more power and prestige (Burton and Goodman 2011). Creating a nurturing environment and being available to listen, talk and offer help and advice are seen as key parts of the support role, and many of the skills and behaviours discussed in the previous chapter are relevant to these staff. Children's parents can find it easier to develop relationships with support staff rather than with teachers, and this can help to develop a collaborative approach between home and school to meet the child's needs (Burton and Goodman 2011).

A large-scale study involving 736 schools in England set out to find out how mental health issues were addressed and how emotional well-being was promoted (Vostanis *et al.* 2012). This revealed that more emphasis was put on reacting to pupils with existing and emerging problems than on preventative approaches. Most of the staff involved in providing support had no specialist training and only 17 per cent of schools reported that they provided counselling and support for their teachers and other school staff. A consistent picture that emerges from the research into mental health within schools is the importance of a socially supportive atmosphere for all staff as well as pupils in a school and that this needs to be part of a whole-school approach (Cooper 2011b; Kidger *et al.* 2010). Peer support and mentoring schemes in schools seem to help to improve the self-esteem and social support experienced by pupils, particularly those who are the victims of bullying (Houlston, Smith and Jessel 2011).

The key role that staff can play in pupils' welfare has implications for teacher-training programmes (Bostock, Kitt and Kitt 2011; Cooper 2011a). It has been suggested that teachers could be supported in developing an 'emotional health and well-being' approach to their work, both in initial training and in on-going professional development (Kidger *et al.* 2010). Kidger and colleagues identified a number of barriers to teachers becoming more involved in pupil welfare issues. These barriers included: concerns that such work would cut into subject-based teaching time, lack of knowledge about how to go about it and teachers' own stress and emotional strain. It has been suggested that such difficulties could be tackled in schools by having clear aims and strategies for emotional well-being work, the provision of on-going training and ensuring support for teachers' own needs as they carry out the work (Kidger *et al.* 2010).

Social support in further education

By its very nature, further education can attract students who are unlikely to succeed without appropriate support being available:

> 'The population is vulnerable. Students between the ages of 16 and 18 will become exposed to drugs. Leaving school is a big transition. Mature students on entering college may find resonances and have to deal with their past experiences of failure [causing] emotional re-stimulation. Coming to college can be an added pressure to their daily lives and some find it difficult to balance their studies and their family commitments.'
>
> *(College counsellor, Leach 2004)*

Further education colleges recruit a number of students who have experienced previous failures, interruptions or difficulties with their earlier school education. One regional study reported that 26 per cent of further education students sampled had experienced intrusive emotional or psychological problems in the current academic term (Schools Health Education Unit 2002). In addition, mental health service users may be encouraged to use further education as part of their recovery programme:

> 'External agencies often see FE [further education] as a useful way back in for clients who need to gain some structure in their lives.

> The college doesn't know about all the students with mental health difficulties who enrol for courses.'
>
> *(Student services manager, Leach 2004)*

Specialised supported education programmes have been set up in some colleges in the UK. However, as the above quote suggests, many further education colleges may find they are seen as a useful resource, but without any formal arrangements with other agencies having been put in place. As counselling services in these colleges tend not to be resourced to the extent that is found in higher education, various forms of social support can be particularly relevant in this context.

Further education can play a valuable role in offering a second chance to people affected by mental health problems to make up for previously interrupted education and to gain a sense of moving on and acquiring new skills and confidence (James 2002; Lewis 2012; Wertheimer 1997). Policies of widening participation are closely linked to the further education sector's role in providing opportunities to develop the skills and qualifications needed for higher education, employment and community participation (Williams 2012). Although potentially positive, the experience of going to college is not always an easy one for students who have struggled with their mental health:

> 'Most of the students are people trying to build up their lives. They are not all at crisis point, but are stumbling along and bring a lot of baggage with them. And then they are put together in an academic environment with lots of others with problems and we expect them to be successful.'
>
> *(GP, Leach 2004)*

Cathie Hammond (2004) conducted interviews with 142 mental health service users who were engaged in community or further education courses and found that they identified many benefits for their mental health. Support from lecturers and from fellow students was rated highly as a contributing factor to their success in education. Although the respondents to this research identified the benefits of gaining new knowledge and skills, they also rated highly the opportunities for making new friends and accessing new social worlds that education offered. Many of those interviewed felt that their mental health had improved as a result of developing greater self-confidence and self-efficacy (personal control and effectiveness) through participation in adult education. Education also offered them a chance to develop a more positive identity and, for some, promoted a sense of purpose and hope (Hammond 2004).

An interesting illustration of how further and adult education can be used to improve mental health came from a collaboration between Northamptonshire Teaching Primary Care Trust and Northamptonshire County Council Adult Learning Service. They developed an adult education programme focusing on well-being, creative expression and healthy living for people affected by mild to moderate anxiety and depression. An evaluation by the Mental Health Foundation (2011) measured the mental health of 256 participants at the start and end of the programme and again at 6 and 12 months after it had finished. The results were encouraging, with an overall increase in well-being and a reduction in severity of symptoms of depression and anxiety by the end of the programme. These improvements in mental health were still in effect a year later. The evaluation showed the importance of social factors, with respondents appreciating being in a community-based educational, rather than clinical, setting. They reported feeling less isolated and, in some cases, enjoying participating in social groups. The input and support of tutors was acknowledged as an important factor.

Students in the further education sector will face some of the same issues as those in higher education although the context is different:

> 'The college has an extra dimension, compared with most university students, that many students live with their parents. This can be a positive or a negative factor. It docs mean that staff often have direct dealings with parents.'
>
> *(Student services manager, Leach 2004)*

The majority of further education students live at home with their families. Many young further education students use families as a source of support (Worral and Law 2009), thus much of what has been said in the previous chapter about support from family and friends will apply to students who are affected by mental health problems. Nevertheless, the college of further education offers an opportunity to access other forms of help, which may help the individual become less dependent on family members for support. Additionally, not all students find their families supportive and some will have problems that have arisen as a result of disturbed family relationships.

As in other contexts, help-seeking behaviour in further education can be affected by a number of factors including shame, stigma, fear and embarrassment, which can deter students from talking about their problems:

> 'Some students with mental health difficulties don't want to reveal or acknowledge their problems. For instance one student could admit to being a heroin user but not to his depression.'
>
> *(College counsellor, Leach 2004)*

This suggests the need for support systems that are available to all students without them having to identify themselves as having a diagnosed (or diagnosable) mental health problem. However, some students are likely to need more specialist support. A psychiatrist working in a children's and adolescents' mental health service pointed out that colleges may experience a significant number of young people with recognised mental health problems who are going through a difficult transition:

> 'Probably half of our clients go on to some form of further or higher education. Community studies show that around 10 per cent of young people are affected by mental health problems, although they may not seek treatment, so there will be many students affected in a college... When the clients move on post-18 they will often still have links with the health systems... Unfortunately the level of support, including psychological support, drops when they enter adult services, so additional support would be very helpful at this stage. Some want a fresh start and might not want to be linked into support services, but it is useful to have a safety net. Even if they don't use it, the knowledge that it is there would be helpful. Having no safety net on entering further and higher education could be quite anxiety-provoking.'
>
> *(Psychiatrist, Leach 2004)*

Colleges will contain students with a range of problems. Some students will have had contact with mental health services, whereas others have had no professional support at all. Some will have short-lived difficulties linked to current circumstances, whereas others will have been affected for some time and will be hoping that education will help them to achieve a more positive situation in their lives. For those individuals with long-term and severe problems, supported further education allows extra help to be put in place to address the barriers and difficulties that might prevent them from accessing, staying in and successfully completing education and training.

The requirements of equalities legislation and the difficulties and concerns raised by staff in further education all point to the need for a planned approach to identifying and meeting mental health needs in colleges. Ian Warwick and colleagues (2008) conducted case studies of such support in five colleges of further education and reported that there were positive examples of support systems for vulnerable students. They highlighted the need for staff training and for developing partnerships with external agencies. There is no consistent approach across the UK to using supported further education as a pathway to improved mental health for service users, but a number of local projects have been developed. Analysis of one such project in southern England found that service users entering the programme with a low sense of 'coherence' (being able and willing to identify and manage demands made by the person's internal and external environment) were able to significantly improve their sense of coherence during the course of an academic year. It was found that peer support encouraged engagement with learning activities and promoted the uptake of staff support and that students reported a reduction in symptoms and an increase in positive mood (Morrison and Clift 2006). As an example of what can be offered, New College in Nottingham provides a 'well-being and mental health support service' with support from specialist staff at every stage from an initial pre-application visit, entry and induction through to studying and taking exams (James 2002; New College Nottingham 2012).

The supported education approach available in some areas of the UK is only one part of the picture. Many students in mainstream further education provision will enter college with, or subsequently develop, mental health issues, but not need or want specialist provision. Although separate supported programmes can be valuable for service users who have intensive support needs, making mainstream education accessible is the preferred route for promoting social inclusion and challenging stigma. Of course, this makes particular demands on teaching staff:

> 'Academic staff do find support difficult, for instance suicidal expression is very frightening to tutors... Tutors can also

become over-involved. Widening participation raises the issues of boundaries for the tutors. Students may reveal difficult issues to their tutor, but where does the person take it?'

(College counsellor, Leach 2004)

In contrast to staff working in health and psychotherapeutic services, academic staff do not have the specialist training, supervision and referral networks that can support working with issues of mental distress and disturbance. Teaching staff have a number of roles and they have to be careful about how they manage these:

'There are some tutors who are over-involved e.g. one who gets terribly involved in students' lives and tells them about her own problems. But tutors have other roles like marking and giving feedback on work and that doesn't fit with getting too personally involved.'

(College advice worker, Leach 2004)

Tutors need support to develop successful strategies for meeting these demands. In a small research project I conducted with community and adult education staff (Leach 1997), four main areas of concern were identified: support, integration, information and safety.

Support for the student requires providing them with opportunities to state any particular needs that they may have, being clear about what the tutor can and cannot offer and helping to identify other sources of appropriate support for those areas that are outside of the tutor's remit. Other students in the group were also identified as needing support so as to create an inclusive atmosphere. Support for staff members themselves was also seen to be very important; staff particularly felt the need to discuss the best ways of addressing challenging situations with a sympathetic manager.

Integration of a student with mental health problems within the group was seen as something that staff should try to influence. Use of warm-up or icebreaker activities was recommended, along with making use of small group activities during a teaching session. Working in pairs on cooperative activities was also suggested, but with the proviso that the distressed student should not always be paired with the same partner. It was felt that without such interventions, it was likely that cliques would develop, which would increase vulnerable students' feelings of isolation. At the same time, tutors were aware that some people find it hard to relate to others and that the pace and process of social integration should be handled sensitively.

Issues raised about *information* were closely linked to concerns around confidentiality. It was considered helpful if students felt able to provide information about their needs to staff. Examples included: knowing that a student suffering from anxiety might prefer to sit near the door in the classroom or understanding that a student with depression might have to miss some lessons. Staff felt that they would at times like to share this information with others in the institution in order to best meet the students' needs but were conscious of the sensitive nature of this information. A particularly difficult area was what, if anything, to share with the other students in the group. Many students would be aware that a particular individual was 'different' in some way and tutors felt that their help could be enlisted if there was some open discussion about how that person's needs could be accommodated within the group. Although some students with mental health issues had reached a point where they felt safe to discuss their situation, others would be horrified at the idea. Another question was about whom to contact if they were concerned about the student; this could be a key worker, an advice service or a crisis response team.

Safety was a key concern for staff, who felt that, in a few cases, a possibility of violence existed. Some had certainly witnessed examples of challenging behaviour. Although they acknowledged this was very rare, there was a sense that care should be taken to avoid risky situations. To this end it was recommended that one-to-one meetings with students should not take place in isolated locations, that managers should be consulted and, where necessary, staff should have training in dealing with challenging behaviour. Feeling safe also involved knowledge of the appropriate boundaries in the relationship with students and keeping to these. There was a fear that, in being sympathetic and supportive, a dependent relationship might be created (Leach 1997).

As part of the same research, interviews with a small sample consisting of five mental health service users who had attended adult or further education classes revealed what they had found helpful. In common with the points made by tutors about integration, the social climate of the classroom was felt to be very important. None of the students had revealed that they had a mental health problem.

All reported feeling very nervous at the first class. They began to feel more comfortable if the tutor included icebreaking or similar activities that helped students get to know each other. In those cases where no such activities occurred, the students felt anxious and two of them described how they had abandoned classes because of the lack of a sociable atmosphere. All students saw the tutor as playing a pivotal role in creating the right social environment (Leach 1997).

Developing socially supportive teaching environments benefits all students, including those with specific mental health needs, and an understanding of group dynamics is an extremely useful skill for tutors (Rogers 1986). So, to a large extent, good practice in adult education (creating a positive atmosphere, providing a range of activities and building in opportunities for social interaction and collaboration) makes education accessible to students with mental health problems. Nevertheless, there are times when education staff will need additional support. As discussed in Chapter 2, a key issue in the mental health field is the challenge of different experiences of reality:

> 'What causes most concern are the ones who are unusual. Experiencing things that staff haven't had experience of such as hearing voices etc. It is hard to know what information there is on this topic.'
>
> *(College lecturer, Leach 2004)*

This need for information is something that is often raised by education staff and others who are offering more formal types of social support as part of their job role:

> 'The staff find it difficult to get hold of information from agencies which they need. Staff see the students more than the agencies do, and it would help to have information about the students' background, such as have they had mental health problems before? The trainee may not tell you things before they start, it takes time to build up a relationship and trust. They will get educational information but not more personal details. It would help to build the best programme for the student if they had the information. For example, one student who had had her baby taken into care and that was one of the root problems.'
>
> *(College lecturer, Leach 2004)*

This same issue was raised by a GP who supported a specialist college of further and higher education that had a large intake of students with previous experiences of emotional and mental health issues:

> 'The obvious thing is what do you tell tutors? How much leniency do you give them [students] because of their mental health problems and where does confidentiality fit it in?'
>
> *(GP, Leach 2004)*

There is little published research on the support given to mentally distressed students by further education teaching staff, but one study (Hart 1996) has compared the pastoral skills used by tutors in further education with those of student counsellors. Both made much use of listening skills, but counsellors were more likely to use reflective techniques, whilst tutors were much more likely to use questioning. Tutors rated the value of giving advice more highly than counsellors. The risks of giving advice were mentioned in the previous chapter, but it may be that the advice given by tutors was related to academic rather than mental health issues. The author of that study makes an interesting point; the creation of counselling services in educational institutions may lead to a reduction in the personal support given by teaching staff. The availability of trained counsellors can give the message that any emotionally laden issues are best left to the 'professionals' and, given the time pressures on teaching staff, it would be understandable if they readily referred distressed students on. However, students may be more comfortable talking to someone they already know and may view support from a tutor as less stigmatising than using counselling services.

More research has been carried out into the mental health of students in higher education than those in further education, so the next section has more information than it was possible to present in relation to the latter. However, apart from the fact that many more further education students live at home with their families than those at university, many of the lessons learnt from a higher education context could be applied to further education colleges and vice versa.

Supporting students in higher education

Studies of university students in the UK and elsewhere indicate that they are likely to experience significantly higher levels of anxiety and depression than other people in the general population of a similar age (Bewick *et al.* 2010; El Ansari *et al.* 2011; Houghton *et al.* 2010). Why should this be? It might be assumed that those who are fortunate enough to have succeeded in going to university should be happier than their peers who have not. Research studies have measured a significant rise in self-reported symptoms of anxiety and depression in samples of students tested before and after entering the first year of higher education (Bewick *et al.* 2010; Andrews and Wilding 2004). This decline in mental health seems not just to be about initial problems of transition and homesickness because, for as many as a third of all students, symptoms of psychological distress persist throughout all the years at university and have been reported to reach a peak in the final year (Bewick *et al.* 2010; Houghton *et al.* 2012; Stallman 2010). A study in Canterbury in the UK found that, whilst on average the psychological distress experienced by a cohort of students decreased between the first and second years of university, the proportions experiencing potentially serious levels of distress only fell from 39 per cent to 35 per cent and within this group there was no significant reduction in the degree of distress experienced (Mitchell, MacInnes and Morrison 2008).

Taking the long-term view, having higher education qualifications has been linked to having better mental health in later years (Higher Education Funding Council 2001; Singleton *et al.* 2001). This suggests there is something about the process of going to and being at university that challenges mental well-being at the time. Getting off to a good start at university or college is certainly important. Many university students have moved away from their families and from the social support networks associated with their previous location and are thus faced with having to build new social relationships if they are to avoid isolation. At this time there may be a tendency for psychologically distressed individuals to form lower quality social networks than those who are experiencing higher levels of well-being (Newland and Furnham 1999). It has also been suggested that a student's ability to form supportive networks and to adjust to university life may be affected by personality factors such as neuroticism, extroversion, self-esteem, social inhibition and perceived social competence (Halamandaris 1995). Feelings of isolation and loneliness are strongly correlated with a high score on measures of psychological distress in student well-being surveys (Mitchell *et al.* 2008) and social anxiety about forming friendships features strongly in students' concerns (Gibney *et al.* 2011; Russell and Shaw 2009). These findings suggest that extra attention could usefully be given to helping vulnerable individuals form social relationships early on in their studies.

A number of studies have highlighted the link between financial difficulties, student debt and psychological disturbance (El Ansari *et al.* 2011, Jessop, Herberts and Solomon 2005). One team of researchers has reported that students in debt were more likely to report knowing other students who were involved in prostitution, crime or drug dealing in order to help support themselves financially (Roberts, Golding and Towell 1998; Roberts *et al.* 1999; Roberts *et al.* 2000). Students' elevated levels of anxiety and depression have been correlated with anticipated levels of graduate debt (Stradling 2001). These studies were carried out prior to the introduction of the current student loans system in England, and it will be interesting to see if this makes any difference to students' money management problems, perception of debt and associated mental distress.

Surveys indicate that one of the most stressful aspects of education, as perceived by students, is exams and assessment (El Ansari *et al.* 2011; Mitchell *et al.* 2008). Students' levels of anxiety and obsessionality have been found to increase in the months before exams, whilst levels of depression tend to rise in the period between taking exams and receiving the results (Fisher 1994; Surtees, Wainwright and Pharoah 2000). A lot depends on students passing courses and getting good grades. The situation in which approval from significant others is conditional upon performing well at university can be contrasted with one of the conditions identified by Carl Rogers (1951) for good mental health. 'Unconditional positive regard' refers to the experience of being accepted and liked for who you are, not what you do. It is not surprising that people can become highly anxious when they feel they are only acceptable if they are able to maintain high standards. Although this conditionality has driven some students to great success, there are maladaptive aspects of perfectionism; the experience of positive self-esteem and the avoidance of depression can be tied to a constant need for achievement (Rice, Ashby and Slaney 1998). Academic staff may need to put students under a certain amount of pressure but if this is not balanced with appropriate levels of reassurance and support, some students with issues of low self-esteem or perfectionism are likely to be destabilised by that feeling of pressure:

> 'People's moods can change a lot, e.g. students can feel great when they are complimented by a tutor but criticism has the opposite effect on their moods.'
>
> *(Student, Leach 2004)*

In more informal educational contexts, engagement with adult education throughout life seems to be beneficial to mental health (Laal 2012). Organisations such as the National Institute of Adult Continuing Education (NIACE) and the University of the Third Age (U3A) have been promoting the benefits of lifelong learning in the UK for many years. So it is likely that it is the additional stressors associated with higher education that can be challenging to some people's mental well-being rather than the process of learning itself. Whatever the context in which education happens, it would seem that the benefits of the learning process can be enhanced by employing measures to reduce unnecessary stress and by providing timely and appropriate support to learners.

Colleges and universities have increasingly recognised the importance of providing support to vulnerable students, not only for welfare concerns but also pragmatically to improve retention rates. One study (Wilcox, Winn and Fyvie-Gauld 2005) found social support to be a crucial factor in influencing first-year students' decisions about whether to remain or withdraw from university. Whilst all students may find this time of transition difficult, students who are experiencing existing or emerging mental health problems find it particularly challenging to seek help during this stage in their lives (Quinn *et al.* 2009):

> 'I personally kept my own stuff out of sight as I knew there wouldn't be much support and there are very few who will accept you for who you are rather than as a charity case.'
>
> *(Student, Leach 2004)*

When informal social support is not available or not sufficient to meet the individual's needs, counselling, advisory and medical services are often made available to university students. University students are unusual in having relatively quick access to free counselling services in most institutions. However, there seem to be a number of barriers that can inhibit students with mental health concerns from seeking professional help.

Seeking and getting help

Some students, when they think they may be labelled as 'mentally ill', face challenges of embarrassment and the fear of stigma and social rejection. In my research in the further and higher education sector, staff indicated that it was hard to get students to take up the support available from student counselling services. Students did not want to be seen as needing counselling and, if they did use counselling, many did not want others to know about it. There also seemed to be a common misperception amongst some students that use of university counselling services would lead to them receiving a psychiatric diagnosis that would go on their records:

> 'People are unwilling to seek professional counselling and fear that that they will get a label attached to them and they won't go, especially male students. This is to do with a butch macho image. So if you come across a male student with mental health problems it is difficult to know how to approach them as they may not want professional help.'
>
> *(Residential staff member, Leach 2004)*

Fears about stigma are not confined to the student population, but students can have particular concerns about the impact of receiving a psychiatric diagnosis on their future career prospects. This is one factor causing certain students to be reluctant to use formal routes of support especially if they are on a professional programme such as social work or medicine (Chew-Graham, Rogers and Yassim 2003; Stanley *et al.* 2010).

The stigma and fear of being labelled is one factor that makes distressed students more likely to use social support rather than approaching medical or counselling services. Given that a number of studies suggest that around one third of university students experience relatively high levels of distress (El Ansari *et al.* 2011; Houghton *et al.* 2010; Mitchell *et al.* 2008) and that most students have access to free counselling services, it is striking that only around 6 per cent of students take advantage of these services (Turner *et al.* 2007; Walsh, Larsen and Parry 2009). Somewhere between 5 per cent and

14 per cent approach their GP for support and treatment (Mitchell *et al.* 2008; Turner *et al.* 2007). By contrast, studies of students' help-seeking behaviour indicate that sources of social support are used at a much greater rate.

Friends feature significantly, with studies reporting between 22 per cent and 28 per cent of students who experience mental distress using friends as a source of support (Mitchell *et al.* 2008; Turner *et al.* 2007). A significant number of students still use their family for support with psychological problems: for instance, one study in south east England reported 19 per cent doing so (Mitchell *et al.* 2008). The availability of mobile phone, texting and internet-based communications make this support from family at a distance easier than it was for previous generations of students. However, this technological ability to have frequent communication with family members does raise questions about its effect on the young person's development of their own sense of independence and adulthood. Psychologist Terri Apter (2001) suggests that maturity in modern Western society is achieved somewhat later than the legal age of adulthood and that parents can expect to be providing financial and emotional support even after their 'children' have left university.

Studies in Leicester (Grant 2000) and Nottingham (Wolfson 2001) reported that 54 per cent and 47 per cent of students respectively identified their tutors as a key source of emotional support. Stanley and Manthorpe (2001) found that 35 per cent of academic staff surveyed in one university had experiences of supervising students with mental health issues in the past five years. Very little attention has been paid to the supportive roles of non-teaching staff such as librarians, hall wardens, administrators, security staff and cleaners in the literature. However, the value of their involvement has been acknowledged in relation to identifying students at risk of suicide (Stanley and Manthorpe 2002).

What can social support offer to students?

Students are affected by many stressful factors and having a mental health condition, as well as being a reaction to stressful circumstances, can be another source of stress in itself. Lazarus and Folkman developed a model that links stress and coping styles (Lazarus 1999; Lazarus and Folkman 1984). As not all sources of stress can be avoided, they suggest that an individual's mental well-being depends on both their appraisal of the threat posed by the stressor and ability to deal with that challenge. Social support can play a role in reducing the impact of the stresses encountered in further and higher education and can help students to find ways of coping with them:

> 'I also see, later on, those who haven't made such supportive groups around them. You don't tend to hear about problems from those students who are socially integrated. They probably don't have so many problems.'

> *(Tutor, Leach 2004)*

Although major life events, such as bereavement and parental divorce, have a negative impact on some students, the mental health of many more will be significantly affected by day-to-day stressors such as workload, assessment tasks, financial issues and forming relationships (Robotham and Claire 2006). How these are dealt with can have a major impact on well-being. It is possible that the availability of social support increases the chances of the student taking a direct and practical problem-focused approach to managing stress rather than using the less successful 'avoidant coping' strategies (Bouteyre, Maurel and Bernaud 2007; Chao 2011). Avoidant coping can involve: venting emotions, distraction activities, using alcohol or illicit drugs, trying to immerse oneself in academic work or attempting to deny that certain problems exist or are harmful. Such behaviours tend be unsuccessful in that they take up a lot of emotional energy, may involve risky behaviour and leave the underlying difficulties unaddressed:

> 'The basic one is to avoid the problem by not talking about it. Some also try excessive partying, excessive drinking or throwing themselves excessively into their academic work. Some will avoid other people. They do not want to hear that it would help to talk. They prefer to be in denial...'

> *(Student representative, Leach 2004)*

By contrast, problem-focused coping refers to a process of identifying the source of stress and finding means of changing the situation or adapting to it. Emotion-focused coping (Lazarus 1999) plays a role in adapting to stressors that cannot be changed, particularly by engaging in a process of reappraisal of the situation so as to see it as less harmful or even in a positive light. However, a study of daily hassles, depressive symptoms, coping and social support amongst first-year psychology students in France found that emotion-focused coping was associated with higher levels of depression, whereas problem-focused coping was linked to lower levels (Bouteyre *et al.* 2007).

The significance of the relationship between social support and coping styles here is that higher education students are particularly likely to have their social support networks disrupted by the transitions involved in going away to university. Even students who decide to study whilst living at home may find that former friends have moved elsewhere or have developed new priorities that make them less available. New sources of social support can therefore be particularly important in helping to manage the many challenges presented by university life. Students with higher levels of self-reported social support have been found to have better mental and physical health and felt better integrated with their university than those with lower levels (Hixenbaugh, Dewart and Towell 2012):

> 'Students talk a lot about the support they receive from friends. For example there was one girl in my tutorial yesterday who apologised for yawning so much. She had been contacted at 3am by a friend in distress and had stayed with her until 8am.'

> *(Tutor, Leach 2004)*

Fellow students are an important source of social support. They face many of the same challenges and are likely to be in regular contact with each other. The exploration of friendship in Chapter 3 suggested that friends tend to be made on the basis of similarity in status and shared interests, so it is quite understandable that fellow students, particularly those on the same courses, will form a major source of friendship. However, friendships are also sustained by reciprocity, with both parties making a fairly equal contribution to the relationship. So when a student has a mental health problem that limits their ability to put something into the friendship, they may come to be seen as overly 'needy' and dependent, which may weaken their bonds with others:

> 'I had a fellow student phoning three to four times a week for an hour each time. This went on for over six months…the other student was dragging me down too much and I was avoiding college so as not to see her.'

> *(Student, Leach 2004)*

In such instances, early access to other sources of support may help to sustain existing friendships by providing other ways of meeting their 'neediness' outside of their social group. When a distressed or disturbed student is socially isolated, support from fellow students may still be possible if the institution has recruited students to mentoring or welfare support roles. In my research, one university (a former polytechnic) recruited and trained students as residential assistants and wardens in halls of residence so as to provide a first line of support. Similarly, a much older college-based university appointed welfare officers in each college to look out for vulnerable students:

> 'Mostly they will approach friends first, unless it is quite a confidential matter, then they might bypass friends. Perhaps due to a fear that information will leak out or that seeking help affects your friendships. Sometimes better to leave the friendships unaffected by a concern... In some situations the good friend is too casual, welfare officers are official enough but avoids having to go to the doctors, a good role as a bridge.'
>
> *(Student welfare officer, Leach 2004)*

Many students support each other, and while peer group support can be very important it can also be a mixed blessing. Students can collectively raise anxiety levels as they speculate and ruminate on the demands of coursework and assessments without necessarily coming up with solutions to the problems raised. The availability of internet-based social networking sites increases the opportunities to socialise with others without actually meeting up. However, online forums can also generate anxiety or hostility through reactions to negative postings. An example of this is 'flaming', where certain individuals feel less constrained by rules of politeness and empathy than might be the case in face-to-face encounters and can be quite aggressive to other participants in their comments (Orton-Johnson 2007).

Training in some basic listening skills can help peer supporters avoid some of the pitfalls that can occur in informal interactions with someone when they are depressed or otherwise mentally troubled. Training may also encourage students to raise the individual's awareness of support services and possibly to make their use more acceptable:

> 'There is a lot of stigma around the use of counselling services... Counselling is seen as a sign that you are not coping...it should not

be interpreted as a sign of failure but as a sign that you have found another way of coping... I can see the benefits of counselling and say to others "You are lucky to have the time to get that attention."'

(Student, Leach 2004)

While it is common to talk to friends about everyday concerns and anxieties, when some individuals believe that they may be experiencing a mental health problem they may want to keep their troubles separate from their friendship group and could welcome the chance to use counselling services or other external sources of support outside of their normal social context:

> 'Students who have used the counselling service have appreciated that the counsellors are nice and non-judgemental. They would keep mental health problems quiet from friends...'
>
> *(Tutor, Leach 2004)*

Unlike fellow students, academic and other staff are not likely to be seen as potential friends, so they may be able to listen to students' concerns without worries of maintaining reciprocity and equality within the relationship. Of course, many staff are hugely busy and may prefer to see student welfare as the role of the counselling service or some other agency. Nevertheless, many do become involved in supporting students and this may be down to an allocated pastoral role, a concern to promote student retention or because of their personal characteristics;

> 'I am one of life's chatterers and students come to me and it becomes apparent that it is more than trivial chat. They are trying to raise something much closer to them, which they may not be able to identify...the people I talk to know they will not get counselled or referred, they like to talk to you as an aunt or neighbour, I am sure that students prefer that ordinariness.'
>
> *(College librarian, Leach 2004)*

It is a big step for someone to approach a counselling service about their concerns and, as the above quote demonstrates, the familiarity and 'ordinariness' of a supportive figure encountered in everyday life can be very reassuring. Furthermore, academic and residential staff can play a role, not only in listening to students' concerns but also in encouraging them to engage with other students for mutual support:

'In the students' first year I try to get across to them the importance of forming a good friendship group and encourage them to look out for fellow students who are not coping and to approach me about them. If they do I will discuss whether they should do something about it, whether I should or whether we both should. The best thing for carers is to train others to care too.'

(Tutor, Leach 2004)

Academic and residential staff can also encourage use of other services including student counselling and medical services (Walsh *et al.* 2009). Those members of staff who are involved in running, and sometimes are also living in, the residential facilities provided by universities can become particularly aware of the mental health problems that exist in the student community:

'You could say that wardens are more likely to pick up problems than the hall managers who work office hours. Often problems emerge when students come back from their day when they are isolated and lonely in their rooms.'

(Hall of residence staff member, Leach 2004)

These staff may be the first to become involved in a crisis situation, but can also notice students who have become withdrawn and depressed. They describe various strategies for providing support, many of which centre on listening, giving advice and trying to involve others. Some focus on individual support solutions such as accessing counselling and medical services; others speak of trying to build supportive communities within the hall or college environment. For some staff, the seriousness of a few of the situations they dealt with posed considerable worries:

'The major concern is "Am I doing this effectively?" Especially when you only have half the picture and feel inadequately trained... Mental health is a training issue...not training as a counsellor, but training so I can be better at gauging what the problem is.'

(College staff member, Leach 2004)

Academics have long had a pastoral aspect to their work with students and a number of writers have produced books on the topic (for instance: Earwaker 1992; Wheeler and Birtle 1993) to help them in this role. Universities vary greatly in the way they provide tutorial support. Some of the older ones, especially those on the college-based

Oxbridge model, base much of their teaching on tutor–student interactions. By contrast, many of the newer universities, including the former polytechnics, have large numbers of students studying on a modular basis and the experience can be quite impersonal. In the latter case, any one tutor may have a large number of tutees and contact can be infrequent. On top of this there is an increasing pressure on academic workloads, including the need to conduct research and to get published; as a result many academics may feel daunted by the prospect of providing support to distressed students in general and those with specific mental health needs in particular:

> 'Not everyone is good at personal tutoring. Some don't have the time or the skills and you hear of some students who want to transfer to me because of that. The danger is that you can end up with a long list of people.'
>
> *(Tutor, Leach 2004)*

Whatever the limitations on their time, academics can play an important role in helping students manage their anxiety around studying and assessments. Within the literature on student support, the emotional component of teaching and learning seems to be featured increasingly as an important factor. Whereas previously 'pedagogy' was seen as a purely rational cognitive process, the feelings experienced by learners are now starting to be taken into account (Storrie, Ahern and Tuckett 2012; Storrs 2012). Largely dating from the 1990s, and marked by the publication and subsequent popularity of Daniel Goleman's book *Emotional Intelligence* (Goleman 1996), a number of researchers and writers have argued that success in life is not determined by IQ and levels of academic qualifications alone. 'Emotional intelligence' or 'emotional literacy' seems to play a part in enabling students to complete their studies (McLafferty, Mallet and McCauley 2012), to seek help when necessary (Ciarrochi and Deane 2001) and have the necessary self-awareness and interpersonal skills to succeed in their careers (Brackett, Rivers and Salovey 2011; Goleman 1998).

Research studies on the experiences of academic staff suggests that they need to take account of students' emotional reactions in certain situations whilst being careful not to fall into the role of 'therapist'. Asking students to work in groups can generate anxieties both amongst those who find social interactions challenging and others (mainly high achievers) who may fear that they will be held back by fellow students (Storrs 2012). On certain courses, particularly in health care, social work and psychology, reflective activities may raise uncomfortable feelings for some students, as may undertaking work placements with vulnerable clients (Storrie *et al.* 2012). This is not to say that such activities should be avoided; reflecting back on difficulties in one's own life and encountering the problems faced by others can form useful learning opportunities. However, certain students may find such activities particularly stressful and may need additional support in preparing for and engaging with them:

> 'If I touch on sensitive stuff, I will say that "I am aware statistically that some of you will have experienced these issues." I will say as a statement at the beginning that "I am not doing this to upset you." Normally the feedback I get is that I handle sensitive issues well. I do dread the lectures on self-harm and suicide. I talk it quite gently through with them. Some students have emailed me and said "Can I just have the notes?" and I have said "You just come if you can manage it, but it is OK not to come."'
>
> *(Tutor, Leach 2004)*

Establishing and maintaining caring relationships with all students would seem to create a reassuring atmosphere within which learning can take place (Jacklin and Le Riche 2009; O'Brien 2010). In addition, lecturers and disability support staff could be expected to help make adjustments for students whose work has been affected by the episodic nature of their mental health condition. Indeed, under the requirements of UK equalities legislation, any student who formally declares that they have a recognised mental health condition has the right to ask for 'reasonable adjustments' to be made so that they are not disadvantaged in relation to other students. This does require that higher education institutions create an atmosphere of openness where mental health issues are discussed and students feel that it is safe to disclose their mental health condition (Quinn, *et al.* 2009). Such adjustments do not mean lowering academic standards but rather involve allowing extra time for assignments, possibly arranging separate exam facilities and other measures that may be negotiated with the student.

Teaching and residential staff have to maintain a healthy balance between being approachable and not becoming over-involved in complicated emotional and mental health issues. An understanding of what counselling and other services can offer may help these staff in setting appropriate limits in their supportive roles:

> 'I had students inappropriately sent over by their tutor just because they had burst into tears... This sort of referral is determined by the referrer's ability to tolerate distress and knowledge of what is an appropriate case for counselling.'
>
> *(Counsellor, Leach 2004)*

> 'Whilst some academics go to the extreme of saying "never bring any personal problems to me however trivial", others go too far the other way.'
>
> *(Counsellor, Leach 2004)*

Academic and residential staff in universities have a valuable part to play in providing social support to distressed and disturbed students. To do this well, they need some basic skills in listening and an awareness of what they can do to help distressed students in their role of tutor, warden or whatever. Setting appropriate limits to their involvement will be helped by knowing about other sources of support that the student can be referred to when necessary. However, it is important that referral to a professional support service is not seen as being dismissive:

> 'If I referred a student to counselling, I would treat it as an additional resource. I would keep in touch with the student and let them know that they can come in and have a cup of coffee and a chat, a chance to let their hair down.'
>
> *(Tutor, Leach 2004)*

Conclusion: what social supporters can do in educational settings

Having looked at schools, and further and higher educational institutions, can any common aspects of social support for mental health in an educational setting be identified? Applying the theory and lessons from research presented in earlier chapters suggests there are shared issues across different sectors. In Chapter 4 it was suggested that social support could be seen as having five key elements: friendship, emotional support, constructing meaning, offering advice and giving practical assistance. Looking at the range of potential supporters in an educational institution, it can be seen that some of these elements are more appropriate to certain roles than others.

Teachers and tutors have to maintain a professional boundary with their pupils and students, which makes friendships between them problematic. Nevertheless, staff can take a friendly approach. They may possibly offer emotional support and practical assistance and could help in constructing meaning around certain problems. Teaching staff are very likely to give advice, if only to suggest other forms of help such as counselling or medical or specialist disability services to pupils and students affected by mental health issues. For those individuals with a diagnosed mental health condition that they have declared to their institution, they may be linked up with support staff such as teaching assistants, specialist advisers and advocates. The work of these specialist supporters lends itself to provision of emotional support as well as offering advice and practical assistance. Peer support, particularly from one friend to another, could include all five of the elements of social support mentioned above.

The supportive role of families, although operating outside of the institution, should not be forgotten. Depending of the quality of their relationship with the distressed pupil or student, close relatives may well offer all of the elements of social support mentioned. For school-age children, parents are almost always involved in decisions about their support needs. However, once the student has reached the age of 18, sharing information about support needs between the educational institution and the family has to be considered in the light of that student's status as a legal adult.

The stigma attached to having a mental health problem can affect individuals at every level of education and may mean that they are reluctant to use, or be known to be using, special support services. By contrast, social support can be part of the everyday life of an educational institution and thus not viewed as stigmatising. Notwithstanding the benefits of social support, it cannot alone meet *all* the needs of people experiencing serious mental health issues. Given that social support relationships can break down if the supporter becomes overburdened by the other's troubles and needs, it is sensible to try to ensure that all concerned know their limits and are aware that there are other avenues of support, such as counselling, advice and medical services, that can be accessed. That way, socially supportive relationships may endure through difficult times and will be there to help the individual to maintain their place at their school, college or university.

Chapter 6

Working it out

Support in the workplace

Introduction

Work can be an important source of friendship and social support; people in full-time employment may spend more time with their work colleagues than with their family members. Many friendships are formed at work and, indeed, some people meet their romantic partners there. In turn, social support provides a way of coping with the challenges that work often presents. Of course, work takes many forms, with some jobs involving almost constant contact with other people and others being more solitary in nature or taking place in environments that are not conducive to socialising. Some larger employers facilitate social interactions by providing restrooms, cafeterias and, in some cases, social clubs and sports facilities that are available to staff and their families during evenings and weekends. Many jobs are found through word of mouth and by personal recommendation, so the social world and the world of work are closely intertwined. In this chapter, the links between employment, mental health and social support will be explored with reference to research findings, the views of writers on the topic and the experiences of mental health service users.

Employment and mental health service users

Work is rather like a personal relationship; if things are working out well it can be a source of happiness, engagement and fulfilment, but when things go wrong at work it can cause stress, misery and even mental breakdown. Many service users report losing their jobs after developing mental health problems and, whether or not work stress was the cause of their difficulties, keeping up a job whilst in a severely distressed or disturbed mental state can feel nigh on impossible. Nevertheless, many service users who have lost their job, or who never had one in the first place, would like to work. Once the acute stage of a mental health problem has passed, there is no reason why many service users should not resume their old job or enter a new one, although, unfortunately, the stigma and assumptions attached to mental ill-health can raise a number of barriers.

Unemployment rates in the UK and other Western societies have been consistently high over recent years and the situation for people with a history of mental health problems is worse still, with less than 30 per cent being in employment (Mental Health Foundation 2012). Even when work is obtained, access to professional and other higher-level jobs can be difficult, and service users can find themselves working for low wages well below the level for which they are qualified. Whereas unemployment is usually detrimental to well-being and finding a suitable job can lead to an improvement in mental health, entering poor-quality employment tends to lead to poorer mental health (Butterworth *et al.* 2011). With an increasing pressure to get people off incapacity benefits and into work, it is important to pay attention to the nature and quality of the work opportunities available. There is evidence that most service users do want to work or at least to have a meaningful active role in life (Department for Work and Pensions 2009) but, given the difficulties involved, it is understandable that many feel disillusioned about their chances of success:

> 'Mental Health is…a dead weight when it comes to employment – employers continue to deny people access to work but will use another reason to cover their decision.'
>
> *(Respondent, The Open University survey 2011)*

The challenges and barriers faced by people with mental health problems wanting to work should not be underestimated. Gaps in employment do not look good on an application form and explaining them in terms of mental ill-health is not a comfortable option. Getting back onto welfare benefits after taking a job that did not work out can be time consuming and stressful. The challenges posed by certain conditions and by the side effects of some psychiatric medication (such as drowsiness and problems with concentration) can make it difficult for some service users to offer a consistent level of performance. Some individuals have fluctuating conditions; they can function quite well for much of the time but have occasional periods when work will become difficult to manage. In turn, employers may find it hard to see how they can cope with someone who cannot promise consistent performance:

> 'Fundamentally, I think they don't really want to have to deal with anyone who is in any way "different"; they want you to fit in with what they expect of you.'
>
> *(Respondent, The Open University survey 2011)*

The stigma attached to having mental health problems has been mentioned in Chapter 2, and employers and co-workers are as likely to make negative assumptions about service users as anyone else. One study in the UK reported that 51 per cent of the employers surveyed stated that negative attitudes from co-workers posed a barrier to them employing someone with a history of mental health problems (Shaw Trust 2010). The net outcome is that service users experience discrimination and exclusion in relation to employment (Department for Work and Pensions 2009), which deprives the labour market of their talents and acts as a further stressor on their mental well-being.

Health professionals may assume that their clients are no longer suitable for work and it is not uncommon for mental service users to have been advised against considering employment. In recent years, these attitudes have started to be challenged as the benefits of work for mental health have been recognised. The UK's Royal College of Psychiatrists has produced advice urging mental health professionals to take a more positive and supportive approach towards the possibilities of their clients entering or returning to work (Royal College of Psychiatrists 2013). Similarly, a UK government policy document, *No Health Without Mental Health*, states that employment can be part of the recovery process and sets out the expectation that mental health and employment services in the UK will support service users and employers in improving access to jobs (Department of Health 2011).

Employment and well-being

Work has long been recognised as a source of self-esteem; the reverse side is that unemployment or being told that one is incapable of work is a major blow to self-image, confidence and overall well-being. Unemployed people are at much greater risk of depression than those in work (Harrison *et al.* 1999) and are at greater risk of isolation (Reininghaus *et al.* 2008). Therefore it is important that someone who has experienced mental health problems is not assumed to be better off without work:

> 'My life was saved 30 years ago by a consultant and GP who treated me as a distinct individual and set up a scheme that let me become a senior lecturer, successful single parent, school governor, etc. They gave me responsibility and their support.'
>
> *(Respondent, The Open University survey 2011)*

The benefits of work are often divided between extrinsic and intrinsic factors. Extrinsic factors include the obvious ones of earning an income, status and providing a structure for spending time. Intrinsic factors can be satisfaction with the activities involved, a sense of mastery and achieving something, social contact with others and opportunities for self-development. As already mentioned, not all work has a positive impact, and British psychologist Peter Warr (Warr 1987; Warr 2007) has spent much of his career developing a model of work and well-being. Warr's model is made up of the following elements:

1. opportunity for personal control

2. opportunity for skill use

3. externally generated goals

4. variety

5. environmental clarity

6. contact with others

7. availability of money

8. physical security

9. valued social position.

(Warr 2007, p.82)

This model provides a list of conditions considered to be necessary for mental well-being at work. Warr compares these conditions to vitamins, suggesting that, like some vitamins, certain elements are necessary for health up to a certain level beyond which increases will not do any harm, but nor will they provide any significant additional benefit; this applies to items 7–9 in the above list. For example, an increase in pay for someone on a low income will make a significant contribution to their happiness but, for someone who is already well paid, further increases will have little effect. By contrast, for some other vitamins, there is an optimal dose with consequences for health if that is not achieved and also if it is exceeded. Warr says this analogy applies to elements 1–6 in the list. For instance, a job without variety will result in boredom, but a job with too much variety is likely to be quite stressful. Most of the nine elements listed are fairly self-explanatory and will not be explored in detail here, apart from the concept of 'environmental clarity'. This is perhaps a less obvious feature of the workplace, but is an important concept for maintaining mental health. The term refers to the presence of clear expectations built into organisational systems and in the ways that other people behave, so that an individual worker can know what it expected in his or her role and can predict the consequence of his or her own actions in that environment. Feedback from others plays an important part in providing environmental clarity. Too little clarity can result in feelings of anxiety and confusion. An over-controlled environment can lead to loss of personal control and to feelings of helplessness.

Warr's ideas about contact with others at work show many parallels with other writers' thoughts about the value of social interactions. He identifies a number of benefits of a working environment that allows contact with others. The ability to make friends through work reduces the likelihood of loneliness and isolation. Social contact offers the possibility of emotional support for dealing with difficult feelings and of instrumental support to help address specific problems. 'Motivational support' can encourage an individual's persistence during difficult times when the temptation might be to give up. Social contact also helps people to gain a better understanding of themselves through comparison of their thoughts and abilities with those of others and enables the learning of appropriate behaviours for a particular work setting (this is the process of 'secondary socialisation', which was discussed in Chapter 2). Many work and career goals cannot be achieved in isolation, so the opportunity and ability to work in groups contributes towards success and satisfaction in employment. However, as Warr points out, contact with others is only supportive when relationships are positive; there can be very negative aspects to regular contact with others who are aggressive and hostile (Warr 2007).

Warr's vitamin model suggests that social contact is one of the necessary conditions for well-being at work that needs to be present in sufficient quantity but which he identifies as being harmful if the appropriate 'dose' is exceeded. Of course, individuals vary in how much social contact is right for them and some people may not be able to imagine that they could have too much contact with others. People's personalities vary and, in particular, the extent to which they tend towards introversion or extroversion will influence both how much contact they need and the types of work they are likely to enjoy (Cain 2012). Social contact may not be limited to interactions with colleagues, as some jobs require a lot of contact with customers, clients, patients or the general public.

The nature of the physical work environment, and the arrangement of workstations within it, can significantly influence social connections between employees and affect their well-being either positively or negatively (Halpern 1995). An open-plan office that allows much social interaction is likely to favour extroverts, whereas introverts are likely to find this distracting and tiring. Some studies have reported higher levels of well-being and productivity in work environments with views to the outside world, especially when those views are of plants and nature (Heschong 2003; Terrapin Bright Green 2012). When considering employment options for service users, it is not simply a question of 'can they work?', but rather is a matter of asking what sort of work in what type of environment would be likely to be successful for them.

The role of social support in the workplace

'Work colleagues have been supportive. I have been able to change to part-time working which has meant I have been able to keep my job and they've kept my job when I have been off sick for months – and, of course, colleagues have had to cover when I have been off sick.'

(Respondent, The Open University survey 2011)

Social support in the workplace is valuable for all people in employment as a means of dealing with stress and making their jobs more enjoyable;

it is also one of the components that helps people with mental health problems maintain employment. In practice, these two aspects are not very different, although in the latter case the development of social support may need to be more planned and explicit than in the former where it often arises naturally.

Social support has been recognised as playing a part in buffering against stress and helping people to cope with its effects (Turner and Brown 2010). Stress in the workplace can have detrimental effects on workers' health and well-being whether or not they have previously been diagnosed as having a mental health problem. Understanding of the long-term links between work and health has been informed by the 'Whitehall studies' in the UK, which have investigated the health of thousands of civil servants throughout their careers and even into retirement. The first Whitehall study began in 1967 and was particularly concerned with differences in mortality rates between different grades of staff. The Whitehall II study was started in 1985 and managed to recruit over 10,000 London-based government employees aged 35–55. This study, which is on-going, took a wider focus than the earlier study and includes measures of both physical and mental health (Marmot and Brunner 2005).

The Whitehall II study found that work stress was greater for those lower in the hierarchy than those in higher positions. Although this runs counter to popular belief about top executives being highly stressed, it does fit with theories that a major cause of stress is being faced with job demands whilst at the same time having a low degree of control over how that job is carried out (Whitehall II Study Team 2004). The levels of likely mental health problems in this study cohort, as measured by a score of five or more on the General Health Questionnaire (GHQ), were quite high. The GHQ was first administered to the cohort in 1989 and again in a follow-up phase that ran from 1991 to 1993. The results for men for each phase respectively showed that 26.7 per cent and 20.6 per cent had scores indicating a possible mental health problem; for women the figures were somewhat higher at 33.8 per cent and 25.2 per cent. The main factors associated with having a likely mental health problem were having high job demands and putting in a high level of effort accompanied by low levels of reward. Having the ability to make decisions and use skills were associated with a reduced likelihood of having a mental health problem (Stansfeld and Candy 2006).

Figures indicating that around a quarter of civil servants may have mental health problems might seem quite surprising, and it is unlikely that this proportion would receive a psychiatric diagnosis or become mental health service users. The GHQ results are comparable to those found by Goldberg and Huxley (1992), where between 26 per cent and 31.5 per cent of the general adult population were estimated to be affected by mental health problems in any one year. The same authors point out that only 10 per cent of the same population would have their problems recognised as a psychiatric disorder by a doctor, and only 2.3 per cent would use mental health services.

The report on work, stress and health by the Whitehall II Study Team (2004) draws very clear links between experiencing better mental health and having higher levels of social support from colleagues and supervisors. Those employees whose supervisors were not supportive were twice as likely to have a mental health problem compared with other employees. Support was associated with being able to talk about work problems and being given clear and consistent information in the work setting. Because the study was longitudinal, the researchers were able to identify that levels of mental health problems and sickness absence increased where social support diminished over time. Conversely, an increase in social support led to an improvement in mental health. Interestingly, a similar association was found with the incidence of heart disease, so social support at work would also seem to promote better physical health. Social support outside of work was also found to contribute to physical and mental well-being. Employees who had regular contact with friends with whom they could confide and who received emotional support were more likely to experience positive mental health. For those employees who had poor or negative close relationships, there was a greater risk of mental and physical health problems and increased sickness absence (Whitehall II Study Team 2004).

The Whitehall studies have contributed to, and made use of, models that attempt to capture the various aspects of work that affect mental health and well-being, and it is useful that such a large-scale study provides evidence for the benefits of social support at work. As mentioned in the previous section, psychologist Peter Warr has studied this topic for many years and both social contact and social support feature in his model of well-being at work (Warr 2007). Further evidence for the value of social support at work comes from the social psychologist Michael Argyle (1991). Argyle looked at cooperation in working groups and concluded that job satisfaction is increased when work tasks are organised in the form of a cooperative group. These groups operate various informal rules in order to promote cohesion and to manage the inevitable conflicts that arise. It would seem that an important ability when working alongside others and benefiting from the consequent social support is to recognise and follow the informal rules that exist in the workplace. Any attempt to help service users find and keep employment should therefore include how they can be helped to recognise and make use of the informal social networks and rules of the workplace.

Support into work and employment by mental health services

In the last 50 years, mental health services have significantly shifted how they attempt to engage service users with the world of work. In the days of the large mental hospitals or asylums, the more capable patients were given work within the closed community of the institution, for instance doing laundry work or helping to look after the grounds. In some of these institutions, sheltered workshops were developed and would take on simple assembly or packaging tasks for outside businesses. This work was termed 'industrial therapy' and was promoted by the British Institute of Industrial Therapy, which was registered as a charity in 1982.

Even before the large asylums dating from Victorian times started to close, 'sheltered workshops' had been created outside the hospital environment, the largest provider of these being Remploy. This was a state-run organisation catering for disabled people with a range of physical and mental conditions. As in the hospital industrial therapy units, the work tended to consist of fairly simple assembly and packaging tasks. Other mental-health-specific organisations, such as the Richmond Fellowship, also developed sheltered workshops and some organisations started to offer craft and horticultural activities, selling the resulting produce to the public.

There is little doubt that these sheltered workshops were an improvement on the alternative of spending long hours of inactivity in the cigarette-smoke-filled day rooms of mental hospitals, as they offered something to do and contact with others. However, a combination of factors started to create disillusionment with this approach to providing employment and by 2004 the British Institute of Industrial Therapy had ceased to operate as a national organisation. In 2013, Remploy lost its government funding to run sheltered workshops (Brindle 2013). Many organisations that had previously run sheltered workshops now no longer do so and, if they are still involved in employment, tend to offer services supporting service users into mainstream jobs instead. A number of factors probably contributed to this shift in thinking about employment for people with mental health problems. The mental health service user and 'survivor' movement grew in strength from the mid-1980s onwards and, more widely, the disability rights movement changed thinking about social inclusion. These movements opposed segregated provision and promoted the rights of disabled people to have access to the same opportunities as the rest of the population. At the same time, innovations from countries such as the USA, Canada, Australia and New Zealand led to the emergence of 'vocational rehabilitation', which favoured targeted, short-term interventions to help service users into mainstream work. Increasing state interest in getting disabled people off benefits and into work coincided with these other developments and has resulted in funding being directed at support for mainstream rather than sheltered employment.

The role of social support in getting and keeping a job

Although the old-style sheltered workshops and craft-based work schemes effectively segregated service users into a world apart, they did provide opportunities for social support from other service users and from staff members. Participants could get to know each other quite well, as there was often a core of people who might use the service for a number of years. The more recent individualised and short-term approaches to finding work do not provide this rather comfortable form of social support, which had many of the benefits that peer support can bring, as well as having the drawbacks of not facilitating wider social inclusion and perhaps not supporting users to develop their potential more fully.

Individual placement and support (IPS) is now being widely adopted by organisations offering employment support to service users. IPS grew out of the supported employment approach that developed in the USA. Whereas previous approaches used a model of 'train then place', supported employment used a model of 'place then train'. Central to supported employment and IPS is the role of the employment support worker or, as it is termed in the USA, 'job coach'. This person could be seen as a type of formal social supporter, not becoming involved with clinical issues but, instead, supporting their client's efforts in choosing, getting and keeping a job in open employment:

> 'My standard of work has suffered and I have been forced to talk to my employer and colleagues.'
>
> *(Respondent, The Open University survey 2011)*

It can be difficult to admit to having problems with work performance and support workers can play a key role in facilitating discussion about the service user's needs and in identifying reasonable accommodations for those needs. They can become involved in interpersonal issues, talking to the manager about their clients' concerns, such as feelings of guilt about being less productive than other workers or about having special arrangements made for them (Cameron *et al.* 2012; Hatchard 2008).

A study of UK service users' views on what makes supported employment effective (Johnson *et al.* 2009) identified factors that will be familiar from earlier explorations of social support in this book. Emotional support was seen as important in building self-confidence, sustaining motivation and maintaining a focus on employment. Knowing that the support worker was available to them and was willing to talk through issues was highly valued. Service users felt that a good relationship with the support worker was important and felt that this worked best when they met in informal settings rather than more formal ones such as a job centre. Practical assistance in preparing for work, searching for a job and going through the stages of application and recruitment were reported as helpful. The support worker's role as a mediator between client and employer was also mentioned as useful by a few respondents. These findings suggest the value of understanding how to enact the key features of social support within the role of employment support workers.

There are relatively few studies outside of the USA that have evaluated the effectiveness of IPS but it is an area that is starting to receive more attention in the UK and the rest of Europe. In a study that covered locations in six European countries, including the UK, Tom Burns and colleagues (2007) randomly allocated service users to either the best vocational rehabilitation (train then place approach) service available or to an IPS worker. In each case, IPS was more successful in terms of numbers achieving employment, the amount of time spent in employment and the reduction in the use of mental health services during the time of the study. By contrast, a study set in south London did not find that IPS improved employment outcomes, however this could at least in part be due to specific factors in the local context in which the study took place. There was some evidence of lower levels of health service usage amongst those on IPS compared with the control group (Howard *et al.* 2010). Similarly, Justine Schneider and colleagues (2009) found that engagement with supported employment in the UK resulted in the clients reducing their use of mental health services and calculated that over time this would produce savings that would more than cover the costs of providing employment support.

Employment support need not be solely targeted at service users who are unemployed. There is also a role for supporting job retention and return to work for employees affected by mental health problems. There are now a number of research studies that have explored job retention and how it can be facilitated. Cameron *et al.* (2012) conducted interviews with service users about the factors that helped them retain their jobs. Lack of social support and an uncomfortable social atmosphere in the workplace were major concerns for service users. Fear of stigma and of colleagues' negative opinions or reactions affected self-confidence, while actual unpleasantness from colleagues and managers had resulted in some leaving their jobs. Support workers were felt to play a useful mediating role in these situations so as to improve relationships. To do this, they needed good interpersonal skills. Successful job retention sometimes required a change in working patterns or responsibilities, but an important part was the challenging of stigma in the workplace, either through the education of co-workers and supervisors or through boosting the service users' confidence to tackle the issues themselves:

'I spoke to a colleague looking for advice. I was given time, reassurance and great direction in what steps I could follow.'

(Respondent, The Open University survey 2011)

Social support seems to be a key factor in improving the employment success of mental health service users. In addition to making work more pleasant, good relationships with co-workers will help the individual learn how to do the job efficiently and enable them to access support when difficulties are encountered or when the task involved requires input from colleagues. Support within the workplace is better when it is 'natural support' rather than someone external coming in and marking the person out as different. The role of the employment support worker or job coach can be facilitative but should not be too obvious in the workplace. Research by Melissa Roberts and colleagues (2010) found that developing social supports at work had a positive impact on job retention and that natural supports were more effective than paid support. Respondents to The Open University survey (2011) also valued this type of support:

> 'Returning to work, having an understanding manager and colleagues and being made to feel welcome and valued [helped me].'
> *(Respondent, The Open University survey 2011)*

Another UK study explored the experiences of a group of service users who had succeeded in keeping a job for at least 12 months and compared their experiences with those of a group who had not been successful in maintaining work (Secker and Membury 2003). Again, natural supports within the workplace, chiefly from supervisors and colleagues, played a major part in employment success. This study identified certain aspects of that support as being particularly helpful. Training and support to carry out key job functions enabled the service users to build their skills and confidence in carrying out their duties. Relationships with colleagues were important in sustaining the work during difficult times and in finding solutions to problems. A workplace culture that promoted a relaxed atmosphere, tolerated differences and showed a concern for all workers' welfare was identified as helpful. These supportive aspects worked best when backed up by sympathetic staff managers who showed a concern for welfare, set clear expectations about the work to be done and provided constructively critical feedback on performance.

The view that natural supports are effective is confirmed by research in the USA, reviewed by Ann Murphy and colleagues (Murphy, Mullen and Spagnolo 2005), who point out that it reduces the need for paid support and increases social integration. They suggest that natural supports can be built up by involving co-workers in the processes of hiring, inducting and training service users entering employment. Natural supports are quite simply the managers and co-workers who are in contact with the service user in the workplace. Much natural and supportive interaction goes on in most workplaces and so the aim is to help the worker with a history of mental health problems to join those social networks. The higher the levels of social support in the workplace, the greater the job satisfaction experienced by mental health clients who are supported into work (Rollins *et al.* 2011).

Professional roles in enabling social support in employment

As mentioned in the previous section, there does seem to be an important role for support workers in helping service users find and maintain employment, but that role within the workplace needs to be a subtle and facilitative one. An external support worker standing alongside the service user at their workstation would mark them out as different and would reduce the likelihood of natural support systems developing. However, service users do value having someone to check in with, who they know they can call on in times of difficulty and who may advocate for them when needed. The UK study by Johnson *et al.* (2009) mentioned previously shows that the aspects of the role of employment support worker most valued by service users mirrors at least four of the five categories of social support outlined in Chapter 4. Emotional support, practical assistance, employment-related advice and a positive friendly relationship all featured as effective factors in finding and keeping a job. Although finding meaning was not specifically identified in this study, motivation and confidence-building measures were, and these could be seen as components of finding meaning.

There are many aspects of the nature of workplace social support that are similar to the types of support given by friends and family; an understanding of these and how they can be facilitated are likely to be useful for employment support workers. Other skills and knowledge needed include, but are not limited to: workplace assessment, making workplace adjustments, mental health awareness training, advocacy, negotiation, mediation and networking (Sainsbury Centre for Mental Health 2009). It can be seen that the successful employment support worker needs a broad range of knowledge, skills and abilities and that good interpersonal skills underpin much of their work. In this context, John Heron's (1990) six-category intervention approach, introduced in Chapter 4, offers a model for being supportive that is not confined to psychotherapeutic situations and contains certain aspects relevant to the employment support worker's interpersonal role.

Prescriptive interventions, i.e. those that attempt to direct the behaviour of the individual, would be used very sparingly and as a last resort, but would be necessary, for example, if the client was breaching health and safety requirements or if the employer was not facing up to their obligations under equalities and employment legislation. *Informative* interventions are very relevant to employment support, as they aim to increase an individual's knowledge and understanding of their situation and to help them find a sense of meaning. *Confronting* interventions as outlined in Heron's framework are not aggressive confrontations but instead are deliberate attempts to raise someone's awareness of aspects of their behaviour or thought processes that are holding them back. These are quite likely to be needed when a client does not understand the sort of behaviour appropriate for a particular workplace or where an employer shows a lack of awareness of an employee's needs and rights. *Cathartic* interventions enable an individual to discharge painful emotions; as mentioned in Chapter 4 cathartic interventions should be used with extreme caution, if at all. However, it could be useful for the support worker to be able to hear and respond to the emotional responses of their client and those in contact with them in the workplace. *Catalytic* interventions are focused on promoting self-discovery, self-directed living, learning and problem solving and as such seem very relevant to the progressive reduction of dependence on the support worker as the client or employer become more confident in their own abilities. Finally, *supportive* interventions are aimed at affirming the worth and value of the individual, appreciating their qualities, attitudes and actions and, whether used with the client, their colleagues or their manager, can play an important role in maintaining hope and motivation through difficult times (Heron 1990).

Other professionals can play a role in enabling service users to enter into employment and to have the confidence and skills to engage with the sources of natural support that exist in the workplace. As mentioned earlier, health professionals are being encouraged to be more positive about the employment prospects of service users. In the UK, there has been a major government-backed initiative to give working-age people access to cognitive behavioural therapy (CBT) with one of its aims being to help them gain or retain employment. The Improving Access to Psychological Therapies (IAPT) programme in England offers short-term CBT and has seen over one million clients during the first three years of the project (Department of Health 2012). The official report of this project during this period states that more than 45,000 people who were on the programme moved off sick pay and benefits. Whilst short-term psychological therapy can be helpful, it does not follow that all its recipients will necessarily make a full recovery and is likely that many will want to have access to some form of on-going support. The expectation that mental health problems should not be a barrier to working will require greater flexibility in the timing and availability of support services:

> 'All self-help groups etc. were run during the day time – there seemed little help for someone who was managing employment while still dealing with mental health issues.'
>
> *(Respondent, The Open University survey 2011)*

Although the development of natural supports in the workplace can be very helpful for mental well-being and retaining employment, service users will often prefer not to discuss personal mental health issues with colleagues, therefore it is valuable for them to have access to other support outside the workplace. An employer may accommodate their needs for external support by allowing time off for appointments, but this does mark the person out as different from their colleagues and may lead them to feeling concerned that they are not 'pulling their weight'. So, whether support comes from a mental health nurse, occupational therapist, counsellor, employment support worker, mentor or volunteer befriender, there is a strong case to be made for providing a service that is available after normal working hours.

Alternatives to open employment

> 'I would dearly love drop-in places where one is productive (not having a cuppa and doing a quiz), e.g. art, creative writing, gardening for the community…doing projects in care homes etc.

Projects could either help people express themselves, provide training and/or provide a service for the wider community.'

(Respondent, The Open University survey 2011)

Despite advances in overcoming barriers to mainstream job opportunities, there remains a need for employment-like activities for service users who are unable or unwilling to enter 'open employment' but who would like to be actively engaged with others. Social firms offer one such possibility and, although they are still more sheltered than mainstream work settings, they are often based in commercial or industrial sites and offer services directly to the public or to commercial organisations and thus offer some degree of integration. Social firms have their origins in the American clubhouse movement. Clubhouses offer their members a range of activities, including employment through social firms or through taking on job roles that can be fulfilled by more than one person, thus providing continuity to the employer whilst accommodating the needs of service users with fluctuating conditions (Carolan *et al.* 2011). In the UK, social firms are less likely to be associated with clubhouses and often take the form of social enterprises such as community cafes, horticultural projects or bicycle repair workshops. The aim of such organisations is to raise a significant proportion of their funding through generating business income to pay competitive wage levels where possible. Social firms are prepared to make allowances and adjustments for the mental and physical problems faced by their employees and aim to offer a non-stigmatising environment. This means that they may be able to cope with higher levels of mental-health-related disability than many mainstream employers.

American social work academic James Mandiberg (2012; Mandiberg and Warner 2013) has written of the dangers of assuming that assimilation within the mainstream is always the best goal for all mental health service users. Instead, he argues that there can be strength in having different cultural communities, as has happened with many immigrant groups in the USA, forming a 'patchwork quilt' rather than a 'melting pot'. Where stigma and exclusion in the wider society limit opportunities for development and seem difficult to overcome in the short term, identity communities, such as those based around ethnicity or disability, offer the possibility of developing supportive networks, new businesses and skills in community leadership.

Mandiberg argues that once this development has occurred, members of an identity community are in a stronger position in relation to the broader community, and may choose to move between the two. In relation to employment, this could mean supporting business start-ups by individuals with a history of mental health problems and encouraging the development of social enterprises. Within the UK, Gilbert *et al.* (2013) have similarly argued that social enterprises should sit alongside the supported-employment IPS model, allowing for the diversity of needs that exist amongst mental health service users. The number of social enterprises in the UK employing people with mental health problems has grown over the years but is still relatively low, so if the advantages they offer are to be spread more widely, a case needs to be made for supporting their development.

There are relatively few studies that have evaluated the benefits of social enterprises for mental health service users, but those that have report positive outcomes. One study found that participants in social firms in Scotland gained a sense of belonging and acceptance that supported their recovery from mental health problems (Svanberg, Gumley and Wilson 2010). A larger Italian study found a strong correlation between job satisfaction and the flexibility and social support offered by social enterprises for individuals diagnosed with severe mental illness (Villotti *et al.* 2012). A small-scale Canadian study explored the quality of life of individuals with severe mental illness working in social enterprises and found that the status of being a 'good worker' in the organisation was an important contributor to their well-being. Good social relationships with co-workers and supervisors were also significant factors in their job satisfaction and overall quality of life (Lanctôt, Durand and Corbière 2012). Other alternatives to employment such as volunteering, time banks and social activities will be discussed in the next chapter, but it is worth noting at this stage that the social support components of any work-like activity seem to be an important factor in promoting well-being.

Conclusion: work, social support and mental health

Although there are many factors affecting the employment opportunities of mental health service users, the presence or absence of social support would seem to be a key element in entering and maintaining employment. Furthermore, the quality of everyone's mental well-being at work, whether or not they have a diagnosed mental health problem, seems to be enhanced by social support at work. Within the workplace, natural supports can help with integration, problem solving, stress reduction and the learning of new skills. With the move away from sheltered workshops, there is more pressure on service users to fit in with the demands of open employment, but work settings also need to be able to meet their needs, including those for social support. This more inclusive approach helps to counter previous assumptions that the experience of major mental health problems would render the service user incapable of mainstream employment, but it risks leaving behind some people with complex needs. Social firms and social enterprises offer the possibility of providing a socially supportive work atmosphere in community settings for service users whose current needs cannot be met by the supported employment/individual placement and support approaches that are being increasingly deployed.

Chapter 7

The bigger picture

Communities, social networks
and social support

Introduction

In the previous three chapters, social support has been considered
in specific contexts: family, friendships, education and employment.
These different contexts are situated in, and influenced by, communities.
Communities can be thought of in geographical terms, for instance a
village or an area within a town or city, but they can also be conceived
of as groups of people brought together by shared interests, beliefs and
experiences. In some instances, the term is used to group together a
very wide range of people who may never know each other: 'the black
community' or 'the gay community', but the focus of this chapter is on
the types of community in which people are likely to have some form
of interaction with each other.

Social connections and networks are a key part of community life
and this is an important factor to consider for people with mental health
problems, the vast majority of whom are 'living in the community'.
Particularly because of the stigma attached to mental health problems,
there is a danger that a person who has been assisted to 'live in the
community' will do so only in the geographical sense and not in the
social one. This chapter will explore the links between mental well-
being and social support in the community.

Communities: traditional and modern

The word 'community' may evoke a nostalgic vision of a rural village or an urban row of terraced houses where everybody knows each other, carries out much of their everyday activities and feels safe and supported. Although some such communities may still exist, they probably do not reflect the reality for many people in the UK and other Western societies. Factors such as the need to travel further or move to a new location for work, migration to and from the UK, the loss of small, local shops and the decline in church attendance, combined with the steady growth of technology-based home entertainments, are likely to have changed the nature of community life.

The characteristics of the geographical community or 'neighbourhood' in which people live can have a significant impact on their mental well-being. Factors such as lack of facilities, high density of population, high levels of unemployment and fear of crime in a locality present major challenges to mental health (Ivory *et al.* 2011; Kim 2010). Some local communities are quite impersonal, making it difficult for anyone to feel connected to others in the area. However, very cohesive and established communities can be difficult to join as an 'outsider'. So there can be a range of factors beyond the individual's control that make being part of a community difficult.

'Community' is a very general concept and in practice there is a diversity of 'communities'. Ethnic, cultural, regional or socio-economic differences, rural–urban divides and age profiles all contribute to this diversity, affecting the balance between individualism and collectivism, cohesion and fragmentation and the extent to which communities are open or closed. Individuals often tend to identify and socialise with others who are similar to themselves (Neal 2013; Jenkins 2008), so whilst areas with diverse population characteristics (chiefly inner-city areas) can be quite stimulating and liberating compared with more homogenous neighbourhoods, they may also be less likely to promote socialising between neighbours.

It could be argued that Western cultures place more value on individualism and personal self-sufficiency than do Eastern ones (Fernando 2002). In industrialised societies, the idea of community may still be seen morally as a 'good thing'; various social problems are often described as posing a 'threat to the community'. However, in practice social connections within a local community may be quite loose. The idea that the nature of community life has changed with industrialisation is not a new one. In 1877, sociologist Ferdinand Tönnies published a book in which he suggested that there was a fundamental shift in the way that society and human relationships were organised. The older, agricultural-based society was founded on close groups of people living and working together who all knew each other and each other's business. Tönnies used the German term *Gemeinschaft* to describe this form of social organisation, within which patterns and standards of behaviour were largely regulated by the moral codes and sanctions that existed within the local community. The fast-growing industrial society was typified by a much less personal and more contractual and calculating approach to relationships termed *Gesellschaft*. In this modern form of society, the state and its institutions took on a greater role of regulating behaviour (Tönnies 1957, first published 1877). Subsequent sociologists such as Durkheim, Simmel and Wirth similarly have written about the loss of the old close-knit community, with increasing urbanisation leading to more impersonal but less socially constrained relationships (Worsley 1992).

In the mid-20th century, Young and Willmott's famous sociological study *Family and Kinship in East London* (1962) showed that close-knit and fairly stable communities existed within inner-city areas. They described Bethnal Green as an area where people were born and brought up with their kinfolk living nearby. Personal acquaintanceships and connections through kin led to inhabitants knowing a wide range of people beyond their own family. In many ways, life in Bethnal Green in the 1950s was not dissimilar to rural village life in the previous century. Inhabitants stayed near their families of origin after getting married. They shopped and socialised locally and knew stories about the lives of their fellow citizens in the area.

The same study looked at the circumstances of families who left Bethnal Green to be rehoused in a post-war, council-housing development 20 miles away in Essex. 'Greenleigh' was modern and purpose-built with a much lower density layout than Bethnal Green and with a better quality of housing. However, many of the participants in the research reported that their new town was not sociable and there was a culture of 'keeping themselves to themselves'. The authors speculated that the reason for this unfriendliness was the loss of direct contact with kin and that this loss was made up for by a focus on the status of the home, as judged by material standards. This was considered to make the residents more competitive and status conscious at the expense of developing personal relationships (Young and Willmott 1962). The individualised lifestyles found in 'Greenleigh' can be seen to be replicated in many housing developments, both public and private, since the end of the Second World War.

More recently, a comparison of experiences of neighbourliness in two UK wide surveys, conducted 28 years apart, found that people in the general population are less likely than before to know their neighbours. Whereas in 1982, 59 per cent of respondents said that at least one of their neighbours often called in for a chat, by 2010 this had dropped to 22 per cent (Mayo 2010). The same study found that the average number of neighbours known by name had dropped from 13 to 7. The loss of everyday social support experienced by people affected by such changes is likely to have a negative impact on their mental health. Authors such as Frank Furedi (2004) have suggested that the rise in numbers of people seeing themselves in need of some form of therapy reflects, in part, a move away from community solidarity to the individualisation of experience and a developing sense of personal vulnerability.

Given the apparent decline in communality in everyday life, is the concept of 'community' still of any relevance to our understanding of social relationships, social support and mental health? According to sociologist Richard Jenkins (2008), community still has a symbolic presence in people's consciousness; many individuals can identify with a community and can be identified by others as belonging to it. These days, community membership is on the basis of perceived shared interests and may or may not be tied to a specific geographical area. In associating themselves with a particular community, individuals can present themselves to others in ways that symbolise a sense of collectivity. So, for example, a football team's supporters will wear shirts, scarves and hats in their team's colours to emphasise their solidarity in supporting that team. However, Jenkins suggests that, in the modern social context, they may do so without necessarily abandoning certain aspects of themselves that make them different from other members of that community. The seemingly united football supporters will be drawn from different backgrounds and have a diverse range of interests.

With some exceptions, belonging to a village or a part of a town or city is not now the main affiliation for many individuals in the UK or in other countries such as the USA. American sociologist Zachary Neal (2013) has a particular interest in the social relationships associated with city life and has concluded that the most useful way to understand these relationships is in terms of networks. Networks are formed of the observable interactions between people and are more specific and thus easier to map than the vaguer notion of community. Neal identifies two characteristics of social networks as important in terms of receiving support: size and density. People with larger networks have more people to call on and can spread requests for help quite widely. A dense network is one in which there are many links between members, so that many of the people that an individual knows also know each other. By contrast, in a loose-knit or sparse network there are fewer connections between different members. A dense network is likely to lead to more of a sense of community and a greater level of social support.

Social networks, social support and mental health

A key aspect affecting the amount of social support available within a network is the degree of reciprocity in relationships. When many of the relationships in a social network are reciprocal, and doing a favour for someone tends to result in them returning the favour, if not immediately then at some point in the future, there can be a spirit of mutuality and of a sense of obligation to help each other out. If relationships are not reciprocal and favours are not returned, there will be uncertainty about whether or not help will be available in times of need (Neal 2013). Considerations of reciprocity link the social network approach to social exchange theories of human behaviour (Cook and Whitmeyer 1992). These theories suggest that the exchange of goods, information, favours, etc. are the social glue that binds people together creating ties through a sense of mutual obligation.

Although social exchange theories could make social relationships seem very self-interested and coldly calculating, in practice, individuals can enjoy relating to each other in the moment without necessarily maintaining a social balance sheet. It is in the longer term that a lack of reciprocity between two or more people can lead to a breakdown in their friendship (Allan 1989). That said, there are certain situations where (often unspoken) social 'rules' dictate that each person should make a roughly equal contribution in the immediate situation and not just over the long term. One example of this would be shared tasks in work contexts where colleagues are expected to 'pull their weight'. Another particularly strong convention is in the social situation of a group of friends going for a drink where everyone in the group would be expected to buy a round of drinks (Fox 2004). Although individuals may appear to have the personal freedom to flout such rules or conventions, the consequences can be significant in that they may become socially isolated, something that many people would go to some lengths to avoid. Expectations of reciprocity can pose problems for some individuals experiencing mental health difficulties, both practically in terms of perhaps not being able to afford to pay for a round of drinks, and emotionally if they need more support from others than they are able to give back at that time in their lives.

Rather than focusing on geographical communities alone, an understanding of social networks in modern urban life may help people with mental health problems to benefit from greater social participation and social support. The local neighbourhood may offer some possibilities for building social interactions and relationships, but for many people their social networks now extend beyond this immediate geographical location. Unlike the residents of Bethnal Green studied by Young and Willmott (1962) in the 1950s, many modern, urban dwellers have connections with people from different parts of the city or beyond (Neal 2013). In recognition of this changing nature of community and the importance of social connections for the well-being of everyone in society, the UK's Royal Society for the encouragement of the Arts, Commerce and Manufacture (RSA) launched a five-year project to map and develop social networks across a range of communities in England in 2010. This approach identifies social networks, rather than purely geographical communities, as a useful focus for understanding how people connect with each other (Rowson, Broome and Jones 2010).

Social networks can be observed and mapped as patterns of relationships for a range of individuals, thus providing a more specific focus for attention than the more general concept of community. This is not to say that the notion of community is irrelevant, as it does provide a shorthand way of referring to a geographical locality or to a number of people with shared interests. However, a community in this sense will contain a number of social networks, and a social network may link people who are situated in different communities. Urban social networks tend to be larger than rural ones. Family members still feature in urban networks but less strongly than in rural ones because cities offer opportunities to interact with more people through closer physical proximity, contact at work and belonging to various organisations. In urban communities, people are more likely to form networks with others who are similar to them and are at the same stages in their life-course. However, urban settings also increase the opportunity to meet and get to know people from diverse backgrounds. Urban networks tend to be less dense; more people may be known, but fewer of a person's friends know each other compared with those in rural networks. This lack of density can lead to a more impersonal experience of urban living but also offers greater freedom from the relatively conservative norms and expectations of rural communities (Neal 2013). Hence differences of sexual orientation, ethnicity and indeed mental health status may be less significant in terms of choice of lifestyle in an urban rather than rural environment.

Another aspect of modern social networks is that physical distance is less of a constraint to interaction than it used to be. The internet offers many opportunities for people to connect online with each other, regardless of whether they ever have had, or ever will have, face-to-face contact. Some of these online networks mainly connect people who already know each other socially, whilst others are based on finding people with common interests, which can include shared experiences of being diagnosed with a mental health condition. The research on the effects of connecting with others using online networks does not as yet provide a clear picture as to how helpful it is, but the topic is generating increasing interest. There are concerns about how time spent online detracts from direct physical social contact with friends and family (Kang 2007). The impact of unpleasant online behaviours such as 'trolling' and 'cyber-bullying' can be very detrimental to mental well-being (Langos 2012). On the other hand, there is some evidence of the positive effects of receiving social support online (Nabi, Prestin and So 2013). It would seem that online contact can lead to less inhibited interpersonal behaviour because the social norms that regulate face-to-face interactions are less powerful. The internet may be a useful networking tool but one that needs to be used with caution.

Compared with traditional, close-knit communities, modern social networks could provide a wider range of opportunities for someone affected by mental health problems to make social connections. However, research by Sani *et al.* (2012) suggests that social contact is not enough by itself to bring about improved levels of mental health; it also has to have personal meaning for the people concerned and this may well involve their self-identification as being part of a group. Meaningful relationships with others who share similar values and outlooks on life are the building blocks of social networks in which people feel a sense of belonging. In turn, that sense of group membership can foster relationships based on trust, respect and mutual support, which help to counter feelings of anxiety and depression.

Merely living in the same area as other people does not seem to be enough to develop meaningful social connections; relationships tend to be built by putting time and effort into shared interests. To this end, membership of clubs and societies, religious and other organisations can help to build social networks. Joining in a range of activities may be beneficial, as people who encounter each other in more than one context are more likely to connect with each other (Neal 2013). So it would seem that social support can be built by becoming involved in a range of activities that involve contact with others. However, the difficulties in relation to social exclusion faced by individuals who have had a prolonged period of mental distress should not be underestimated. An understanding of the barriers they face is important in the process of challenging discrimination and promoting social interactions.

Social exclusion, inclusion and mental health

Social support from families, friends and community sources can be seen as one of the pillars that supports social inclusion for people with mental health problems. However, it is not sufficient in itself and there are other pillars that also need to be in place (Phillips 2006; Secker 2009). The political and legal systems need to protect the rights of people with mental health problems so that they have access to the goods, services and opportunities available to other members of society. The labour market needs to be flexible and responsive to their needs. The welfare state has to be able to provide income for those who cannot work and offer services that meet their health and social care needs. When an individual is failed by one of these pillars, the other systems need to be available and adequate to compensate. For instance, someone who cannot enter the labour market has to have other means to obtain food, clothing and shelter; someone who has become socially isolated is likely to have an increased need for professional support. For people with mental health problems, often one or more of these pillars is weak; in the worst-case scenario, all of the pillars fail the person, resulting in severe social exclusion.

As mentioned in Chapter 3, social inclusion can be a problematic concept. Social inclusion and social exclusion are not necessarily opposites of each other, and while challenging exclusion can improve lives, there is a danger of inclusion being defined in a limiting and even coercive way (Spandler 2009). Much of the argument here comes down to choice; can the person affected by mental health problems follow the paths to greater social inclusion that they want to take? In Canada, where a similar policy to the UK's has been followed in moving away from hospital to community-based care, community-focused research identified some key barriers to community participation. Leaving a protected and relatively predictable environment raised anxieties for service users about how they would cope in the community. The continued existence of stigmatised attitudes amongst the general public led to uncertainty and concern about how service users would be treated. Financial limitations made it difficult to access transport and to participate in activities. Financial constraints on mental health organisations limited their ability to provide support for community integration (Nelson, Lord and Ochoka 2001).

The same study also noted that personal factors such as diminished self-confidence and social awkwardness posed difficulties for social integration (Nelson *et al.* 2001). Depressed or anxious thoughts, feelings of being disassociated from reality, paranoia and fear can all make it difficult to engage with community life. Similarly, the side effects of some psychiatric medications, particularly those of drowsiness and lethargy, can be a limiting factor. However, it is important to recognise that, as mentioned earlier on in this book, stigma and labelling still present barriers to participation for a significant number of people who have used mental health services. There are therefore both internal personal and external social and political factors that need to be considered when trying to address social exclusion.

On average, people with mental health problems are likely to have more restricted social networks than those without such problems (Howard, Leese and Thornicroft 2000). One UK study looked at the social networks of former long-stay inpatients after 12 years of living in supported community accommodation (Forrester-Jones *et al.* 2012). Members of this group had, on average, a network of 23 people who they knew, a third of whom were fellow service users and another third were staff or volunteers in mental health services. The majority of respondents said that their 'best friends' were people that they had got to know as fellow service users. Overall, family members made up 14 per cent of the network, while friends and social acquaintances not connected with mental health services constituted just 13 per cent, which represents about two to three people for each service user. These figures show a larger social network than might be the case for those with a similar background who have not had such a long period of living in supported accommodation. Even so, they are considerably smaller than the network size of up to 150 or so people that is considered average for members of the general adult population (Roberts and Dunbar 2011). What is also striking is how few people were known outside of a mental health context.

The social networks available to someone with a history of mental health problems can be different from the spread of connections of those who have not experienced such problems and, although potentially supportive, these networks may be less powerful and influential in terms of opening up new opportunities for work, social life or political engagement. There is a wide spectrum of mental health problems and they vary in the degree of impact they have on each individual; it is those with the most severe and enduring difficulties that are most likely to feel the full impact of social exclusion. That said, even people with less severe problems may be affected to some extent by disempowerment and exclusion.

That current and former mental health service users derive much of their social contact and support from others with similar experiences presents advocates of social inclusion with a dilemma. On the one hand, it is widely reported that the most empathetic and reliable support comes from others with lived experiences of mental health problems; this also fits with a sociological understanding that friendships most commonly arise between people with similar background and of similar status (Allan 1989). On the other hand, this can be seen as a form of 'ghettoisation' that deprives service users of a 'normal life'. Restricted networks can deprive service users of the social, economic and cultural benefits that accrue from having contact with others who could be useful in obtaining work or accessing social and other mainstream opportunities (Social Exclusion Unit 2004). In my own experience, there are differing opinions about this issue amongst service users themselves. Some actively identify and involve themselves with service user and survivor organisations, whilst others are very concerned for this not to be a key part of their identity.

Drawing on the experience of ethnic minority communities in the USA James Mandiberg and Richard Warner (2013) suggest that it can be useful to seek support within an oppressed minority community in order to have the strength to face the challenges posed by the wider community. In the context of ethnic groups, this has often involved living in one area of a city and building up businesses and civic and voluntary associations there. This then has provided opportunities for members to develop business and leadership skills, which have helped them to relate to the wider and dominant community. The authors suggest that, although there are not yet any mental health 'identity communities', where specialist housing, business and other organisations are grouped together, there are elements of these in the form of housing enclaves and social enterprises run by service users that could pave the way. Although this is an interesting idea, it is untested and could raise difficult issues of increasing the segregation that the closure of the old asylums was supposed to counter.

Involvement in mental health service user or mainstream social networks is often presented as a dichotomous choice, but it may be that service users could benefit from membership both of social networks that are specifically mental health focused and others that are not. One way of considering how social networks might offer such choices is to look at the concept of 'social capital'.

Social capital, social support and mental health

By the year 1900, the term 'social capital' was being used by economists to describe goods that were required to produce other goods, for example a factory building and the equipment within it. This productive capital was distinguished from 'private' or 'acquisitive' capital such as the savings and valuable items held by individuals (Fetter 1900). In more recent times, 'social capital' has become a way of describing the advantages that can be gained by being connected to other people and from accessing their knowledge, skills and the material and non-material resources they have accrued (Bourdieu 1986). However, there is on-going confusion about the exact nature of the concept and how it can be measured (Phillips 2006; Webber, Huxley and Harris 2011).

French sociologist Pierre Bourdieu (1986) viewed social capital as transcending geographical location, being based in a durable network of personal relationships, providing members with potential access to the economic and cultural capital possessed by other members of the same network. The amount of social capital available to an individual is determined by the size of the network and the quality and quantity of the resources (of whatever type) possessed by fellow network members. Bourdieu described the gains that could come from access to social capital as not just material but also symbolic, which would include feelings of friendship, respect, self-esteem and enhanced cultural and social status. In Bourdieu's formulation, social capital, unlike money in the bank, cannot be stored and left alone until needed; rather it involves a process of continuous exchanges wherein members reaffirm their recognition of each other as belonging to the same group.

American political scientist Robert Putnam (1995, 2000) brought the social capital concept to a wider audience. Putnam was interested in civic engagement, as evidenced by such behaviour as turning out to vote in elections and attending public meetings concerned with education and other areas of public interest. He was concerned that, in the USA, there seemed to be a steady disengagement from civic activities, representing a move from a collective to a more individualistic approach to life. This author also charted a decline in contact with neighbours and a decrease in amount of trust expressed in others. However, at the same time, an increase in non-local friendships was noted. Putnam used the term 'social capital' to refer to the existence of networks, norms of behaviour, and social trust that enable people to work together for their mutual benefit. He saw norms of trust and reciprocity being fostered by civic engagement and the process being one of a virtuous cycle in which successful collective action encourages a community spirit, which in turn makes further collective action more likely.

Neither Putnam nor Bourdieu were looking specifically at the significance of social capital for people with mental health problems, but there have been increasing numbers of subsequent attempts to do so by others. The linking of social capital to mental health is complicated, as there are potentially so many aspects to the concept and the results of research in this area so far are rather inconclusive (Webber *et al.* 2011). It seems easier to find evidence for the benefits of some of the features that make up social capital rather than for the concept itself. For instance, one study (Chappell and Funk 2010) found no support for the thesis that social capital or any of its components (social participation and trust) had a direct effect on health outcomes. However, trust was judged to have an indirect benefit for mental health mediated through feelings of self-efficacy and perceived emotional support. Another study (Giordano and Lindström 2011) reported a stronger association between trust and better mental health. Similarly, De Silva *et al.* (2005) conducted a meta-analysis of quantitative research exploring the evidence for a link between social capital and mental illness. They concluded that there was insufficient evidence to support specific social-capital-based interventions to address mental ill-health, but felt that there was some scope for looking at developing the role of trust in social relationships in order to raise levels of mental health.

Some writers have warned against assuming that all social capital is beneficial for mental well-being. Social capital is a quality of defined social networks and there are often pressures for conformity within those networks. Criminal gangs are examples of groups that have strong norms that can persuade members to take part in activities that are detrimental to themselves and others (Neal 2013). There are also boundaries to network membership, meaning that there are criteria that exclude those who do not fit the dominant norms. Too much social capital may limit the diversity that can be tolerated within a social network (Wakefield and Poland 2005). Another issue is that a very cohesive social network, particularly in low-income groups, can act as a drain on certain members' resources; extensive social connections may carry a wider set of obligations than a looser network

(Moore *et al.* 2009). Furthermore, not all social capital is equal and those with access to high levels of social capital find it easier to acquire more and to move between different social networks that operate in powerful ways. Social capital can be a powerful force in preserving the status quo, which can work against the interests of marginalised groups such as people with mental health problems (Wakefield and Poland 2005).

A distinction can be made between bonding and bridging capital, the former being a property of networks of people who have similar interests and circumstances in common, whereas the latter refers to linkages across different groups, often in relation to an issue of shared concern (Geys and Murdoch 2010). As mentioned in the previous section, service users often find the most supportive networks to be those of other people who have been through the same experiences. This could be seen as an example of bonding social capital that is supportive, but it lacks the opportunities provided by bridging social capital to access jobs, political influence and other social and economic benefits.

Social work academic Jerry Tew (2013) suggests that there are a number of forms of 'capital' that need to be acquired in order to experience recovery from mental health problems. He groups these under the title 'recovery capital' comprising: economic capital, social capital, identity capital, personal/mental capital and relationship capital. Tew's approach mirrors the research on community integration by Geoffrey Nelson and colleagues (2001) in Canada that identified that a combination of personal empowerment, community inclusion and social justice factors were required by service users for a satisfying and valued life in the community. Tew sees recovery as a process that has both personal and social elements to it. He points out that access to capital is only part of the story; the person concerned also has to be motivated to access and use it, so it would be a mistake to focus either solely on the individual or the community when looking at ways of promoting recovery.

Mental health services tend to focus their attention on the individual's problems and, although there has been a major move towards treatment in the community, it is beyond the remit of most professionals to work with the wider community in order to facilitate integration. The whole process of diagnosis, labelling and receiving psychiatric treatment can lead to the individualisation of problems and feelings of vulnerability and dependence (Link and Phelan 2010). Even in the field of social work, there has been a narrowing of focus onto the individual and their problems rather than broader approach that takes the social context into account (Tew *et al.* 2012). Where work on participation and integration does take place, it tends to depend on piecemeal initiatives taken by the voluntary sector (Fieldhouse 2012). It would seem that if service users are to benefit from the social networks available in their community, there needs to be a greater focus on developing that community's capacity to be accepting and supportive.

Conclusion: socially supportive networks

Social support can play a key role in enabling anyone affected by mental health problems to use and benefit from social networks and social capital. As previously defined in this book, social support has a number of aspects: friendship, emotional support, constructing meaning, practical advice and material assistance, all of which can help in accessing social networks in the wider community. Social support is also a product of social capital in networks, so improving service users' access to social capital should also increase the social support they are able to give and receive. Nevertheless, the role and nature of social capital is disputed and it is possible that, if it does have value, it may be more effectively engaged with at a community level rather than at an individual level (Chappell and Funk 2010). So social support may be the means by which individuals develop their capabilities, whilst social capital indicates the collective strength of a network of individuals. The next chapter will look at ways of working at both the individual and the community level to enhance social support for mental health.

Chapter 8

Making it happen

Introduction

Social support would seem to play an important part in improving the quality of life for all members of society. To a large extent, it occurs naturally in the interactions between relatives, friends, neighbours, colleagues and others encountered in everyday life. However, many people with experience of mental health problems report feelings of isolation and loneliness, and research suggests that they tend to have smaller and more limited social networks than other people. So who could be involved in enabling greater access to social support and what sort of actions might help? This chapter will look at some possibilities for engagement by health and social care practitioners and others concerned with the social issues faced by people who experience mental health problems.

The changing policy context

In the UK and many other countries, there has been a growing concern that the provision of clinical mental health services alone cannot address the wide range of issues faced by people with mental health problems. For instance, recent policy documents for mental health in England have included concerns about social exclusion, employment, housing, discrimination and stigma and have stated that stronger social relationships should be an outcome of new decentralised ways of providing mental health services (Department of Health 2011, 2014). Personalisation of health and social care has become a key policy focus in the UK, although the resource constraints faced by public services create some doubts about how effective this can be in practice (Community Care 2013).

The provision of personal budgets in the social care and health sectors is part of the new policy initiative. Personal social care budgets were piloted in England from 2005 (Glendinning *et al.* 2008) and rolled out more widely in 2009. Personal health budgets, at the time of writing, are about to be more widely implemented following trials in a number of pilot sites in England (Alekeson and Rumbold 2013; Forder *et al.* 2012). The guidance for these budgets states that they have to be used for activities that enhance well-being and this is determined by a planning process in which the recipient comes up with a care plan in partnership with a healthcare professional, social worker or care manager. It is possible that these two types of budgets will be brought together to create integrated individual budgets for some individuals in the future (Alekeson and Rumbold 2013). In Wales and Northern Ireland, 'self-directed support schemes' are being introduced (Brindle 2012; Centre for Independent Living NI 2011) whilst in Scotland personal budgets are being made available but service users can still opt for local authority provision (Samuel 2012). The introduction of personal budgets has led to the emergence of case management and brokerage services that can work with service users to determine how they spend their budgets and help them manage the monetary aspects, including the employment of their own care assistants (Hammond 2012).

It remains to be seen how much freedom recipients will have in choosing how to spend their personal budgets. There are concerns about how to ensure the quality and safety of services or activities that have not been approved by the NHS (Alekeson and Rumbold 2013). There is also apprehension that, as these budgets have to be paid for out of existing health and social care finances, there will be difficulties in finding the resources to employ the professionals needed to support the planning and coordination of the care plans that underpin their use (Glendinning *et al.* 2008). Despite these constraints, an evaluation of the personal health budgets pilot in England found some evidence that they were particularly cost effective in meeting the needs of people with mental health problems (Forder *et al.* 2012). Social care budgets have been used by a variety of disabled people, including people with mental health problems who were more likely to use them to access leisure activities than other groups (Glendinning *et al*. 2008).

From a social support perspective, those involved in supporting people with mental health problems could usefully consider how personal budgets could be used to build supportive social networks. If the trend towards providing personalised services and budgets continues, there will be a need to choose between different options, for instance: having individual therapy such as CBT, attending a support group or accessing mainstream activities such as a joining a gym or a social club. In this situation, there may be pressure to provide evidence of the positive mental health outcomes from engaging in different activities. Unfortunately, the benefits of social activities tend not to attract the levels of research and evaluation funding associated with large-scale clinical trials in psychiatry or, to a lesser extent, in psychology. Nevertheless, there is a growing body of evidence that might support the case for funding social engagement. On financial grounds, it has been suggested that personalisation could save local authorities money on their health and social care budgets by increasing the amount of unpaid support that could be accessed by service users if personal budgets helped them connect with social networks in the community (Samuel 2013).

Some of the evidence for the benefits of social support was reviewed in Chapter 3 and, although there is no definite consensus on the exact mechanisms through which it operates, there is general agreement that it has beneficial effects on both physical and mental health. Importantly, service users themselves have identified their desire to lead a 'normal life' with all the social interactions that this entails (Bradshaw, Armour and Roseborough 2007; Forrester-Jones *et al*. 2012). The RSA's Connecting Communities project is collecting evidence on the benefits of developing supportive social networks; the results of this longitudinal study will be useful for evaluating the usefulness of community-based interventions (Rowson *et al*. 2010). On an individual level, experiences such as joining a community choir or participating in group activities such as those focused on horticulture or conservation tasks has been shown to have mental health benefits in lifting mood and improving confidence (Clatworthy, Hinds and Camic 2013; Clift and Morrison 2011; Mind 2007).

Social support seems to help across the range of mental health conditions; it is not only people with experiences such as depression and anxiety that can benefit from improved social connectedness and engagement in activities. Studies have reported that these factors can be important in recovery from schizophrenia and other conditions described in medical parlance as 'severe mental illnesses' (Harvey *et al.* 2007; Hendryx, Green and Perrin 2009). Earlier in this book, it was suggested that mental disorder and mental well-being could be viewed as belonging to different dimensions, or to be on different continua, so that it is possible to experience levels of well-being whilst still being regarded as having a mental health problem (Payton 2009). In support of this, there has been research indicating that individuals with severe mental health problems could benefit from interventions and activities that increase their happiness or sense of subjective well-being even if they are not 'cured' (Mankiewicz, Gresswell and Turner 2013). An interesting new approach (Crawford *et al.* 2013) makes a plea for services and policy makers to embrace a more creative approach to improving mental health, seeing it as a process of 'mutual recovery'. By this the authors mean that service users, informal carers and staff who work in services could jointly focus on activities for all that build resilience and provide a sense of having meaningful lives. The authors suggest that this process also requires that the social context of housing, work, relationships and stigmatising attitudes is addressed. This and all of the above discussion about the changing policy context indicate that mental health services should be aware of the need to work beyond traditional boundaries.

Professional roles and social support contexts

The role of the professional in any occupation tends to involve a fair degree of specialisation; this is how expertise is built up in defined areas of practice. In the mental health field the most common specialisms include: psychiatry, clinical psychology, counselling, nursing, occupational therapy and social work. Many mental health professions focus on one-to-one work with service users rather than connecting them with social networks. This is not to deny the value of individual support in a clinical setting for service users where they can talk in confidence away from the pressures and influence of close family and friends. Additionally, many service users may feel the need for medication or some form of psychotherapy to help them cope with difficult issues. However, whatever the treatment intervention used, the service user is going to return to a social context either immediately or, in the case of inpatients, at some point in the future. If this social context is not supportive, it is likely to hinder the recovery process (Repper and Perkins 2003).

As many professionals work in multidisciplinary teams, they have to find ways of working together and integrating their specialisms so that their service users receive the package of support that meets their needs. In practice, this is not always easy to achieve, as resource constraints and differences in approach can present barriers to providing an integrated service (Colombo *et al.* 2003; Leach and Hall 2011). It would seem that a key aspect of providing an integrated service is to look beyond clinical interventions to the social situation of the service user, including an assessment of the informal support available to them and of the stressors that challenge their well-being. Family therapy and family education interventions recognise the importance of the domestic situation of the service user (Carr 2006), but are not widely available and do not address the social situation beyond the immediate family. In theory, social workers are well placed to take this more holistic approach, which encompasses empowering service users in the social context. However, in practice, they may be constrained by the requirements of the mental health system, which can lead to what seems like a subordinate role of conducting risk assessments and ensuring compliance with medical treatment (Tew 2013).

Studies involving service users and their informal carers suggest that there can be problems in moving between formal and informal care. Discontinuities can occur, so that it is not always easy to reconnect with services nor to know what do when a difficult situation is approaching but has not yet reached a crisis point. Similarly, services are not always very effective in helping service users deal with feelings of social vulnerability in their daily lives (Jones *et al.* 2009). Family and friends are clearly very important in service users' lives but professionals can feel constrained in working with them and this does indeed raise some awkward issues. Another difficulty is posed by the limited resources available to provide mental health services. This can push them towards managing the most severe cases, leaving a gap in the provision for people who do not yet meet the thresholds for receiving specialist services.

There are models of intervention for mental health professionals to use when a service user's social systems are in crisis, and these models are particularly relevant to crisis resolution and assertive outreach teams (Bridgett and Polak 2003). Consideration of the social systems surrounding service users is also promoted by British social work academic Jerry Tew and colleagues, who draw attention to the social factors involved in recovery from mental health problems. Their social perspective on mental health identifies some key elements for recovery: empowerment and regaining control over one's life, rebuilding positive personal and social identities and developing connectedness both at a personal and a wider social level. This approach invites social workers to establish themselves in a more proactive role in the mental health field, a role that maintains a focus on service user empowerment (Tew *et al.* 2012).

All professionals working in the mental health field could usefully consider how they might involve service users, carers, other informal supporters and third-sector or voluntary agencies in a collaborative approach to recovery. This subject has been reviewed by a panel of psychiatrists (Royal College of Psychiatrists 2005), who acknowledged that forming partnerships beyond the boundaries of the multidisciplinary team poses a number of challenges. With such a diversity of potential partners, there is more complexity and uncertainty around roles and responsibilities. There is no established framework to guide the sharing of sensitive or confidential information. There is less clarity about who should inform clinical decision-making. Despite these difficulties, the Royal College of Psychiatrists urges practitioners to engage in developing extended relationships that will help address the vulnerable state of a number of service users in the community.

With the advent of personal health and social care budgets, self-directed support and personalisation, there could be a shift in the relationship between practitioner and client. A larger range of options beyond those traditionally provided by mainstream services is opened up. If service users have a greater say in the package of support they receive, practitioners will need to spend more time on giving information and enabling joint decision-making. There will be challenges in doing this, especially because mental health practice has, unlike other areas of health practice, coercive legal powers that can be used if the person is viewed as posing a risk to themselves or others. This potential for coercion raises questions about how truly 'voluntary' service user compliance with recommendations for treatment actually is (Rogers and Pilgrim 2005). Although only a very small minority of service users will be compelled to receive treatment against their will, the fact that it is possible may affect the power balance in interactions with mental health professionals. This means that it may be necessary to pay more attention to developing relationships based on mutual trust and collaboration than might be the case in other areas of health and disability work. This issue also suggests that service users need to be aware of their rights and to have access to advocacy services that can help them deal with potentially disempowering situations.

At the primary care level, GPs could look at 'social prescribing' as a means of improving mental well-being through increased community participation. Social prescribing involves recommending participation in non-medical activities in order to address mental health issues such as anxiety and depression or to help with improving weight loss and physical fitness. The activities are typically based in the community and often run by non-statutory and voluntary sector organisations (Langford, Baek and Hampson 2013). In order to be effective, social prescribing needs someone to take on a coordinating role that includes developing a list of community resources together with an understanding of what types of activities might be suitable for different service users. It is necessary to be clear about the purpose of the referral and what it might or might not be able to achieve and also to collect information about the quality and impact of the activities prescribed. An important part of the coordinating role is to build and develop relationships between the referring agency and those organisations that provide opportunities for engagement in suitable activities (Keenaghan, Sweeney and McGowan 2012). Examples of activities recommended for social prescribing include: structured physical exercise programmes, nature conservation work, artistic, musical and creative pursuits, community education classes, voluntary work, self-help groups, lunch clubs, befriending schemes and employment and debt advisory services (Keenaghan et al. 2012; South et al. 2008). Social prescribing undoubtedly fits well with a social support approach to mental health, but it does raise certain difficulties that will need to be addressed if it is to become used more widely.

By their very nature, the activities prescribed are in the non-medical domain. Many are provided by voluntary associations and third-sector organisations that can struggle to obtain sufficient funding or to find a steady stream of suitable volunteers. If health services are referring service users to these organisations, should they help by making a contribution to their running costs? Many of these small organisations would not be well equipped or particularly willing to enter into competitive tendering for health service funding. Such funding often comes with requirements for outcome measures and monitoring activities that would not sit comfortably with the way these organisations operate. Another concern would be if any limits should be set on how many people are referred to a particular activity? Participation in community activities is desirable, partly because it provides opportunities for service users to interact with people who are not associated with mental health services. If, for instance, a group undertaking nature conservation tasks had a large proportion of service users as members, would it change the nature of the group? These are not easy issues to deal with but will need to be considered when setting up a social prescribing scheme.

Whether encouraging engagement in community-based activities through the use of personal budgets, social prescribing or other ways of care planning, mental health practitioners need to consider both the social and personal aspects involved in the process. At the social level, the group or organisation providing the activity needs to have a reasonably welcoming and inclusive culture. On the personal level, the individual service user may feel considerable anxiety about entering a new social situation and may need support in developing confidence around social interactions. Some writers have suggested that programmes of social skills training could be beneficial for some service users (Argyle *et al.* 1974; Meltzer *et al.* 2013). Other possibilities include (where available) volunteers acting as individual befrienders or employed staff providing personal support to bridge the gap between being isolated and having the confidence to engage in group activities. Support Time and Recovery (STR) workers, many of whom have personal experience of mental health problems, have been recruited in the UK to provide this more informal type of support

(Huxley *et al.* 2003; Huxley *et al.* 2009). It seems that there are a number of ways for mental health professionals to work with others to address the social needs of their clients and that engaging with local communities is an important part of this process (Fieldhouse 2012).

Enhancing social support: community development work

In recent years, there has been a growing interest in applying a community development work approach to the mental health context (McCabe and Davis 2012). Community development had its origins in work with local communities faced with multiple aspects of deprivation and differs from social work in its emphasis on dealing with social problems collectively (Gilchrist 2004). It is possible that the contested nature of mental health problems and the bad press associated with the early days of 'care in the community' have restricted the use of community development in the mental health field, although there are some recent examples of this approach being adopted (Carpenter and Raj 2012).

Community development work builds and strengthens social networks and thus enables the creation of bonding and bridging social capital. The availability of social support and the sense of belonging that arises from this are potentially beneficial to the mental health of all community members as well as those who have specific mental health problems (Seebohm and Gilchrist 2008). Community development workers can work with communities to reduce the stigma of mental health problems by involving service users in public awareness and education events, which make it easier to talk openly about mental health issues. Other interventions include: helping residents identify unmet needs, supporting the creation of mutual self-help groups, introducing individuals to existing community groups and helping groups to work through difficult times. Community development workers have also been able to play a role in connecting marginalised individuals and groups with mental health and other support services (Seebohm and Gilchrist 2008).

Community development can play a role in highlighting the relationship between inequalities and mental health. A pioneering project in a deprived community in Glasgow, Scotland, has been developed through community-organising and community-building activities. Here, some of the most marginalised people in the community have been empowered through a range of measures including support groups, anti-stigma work and participation in community arts (Quinn and Knifton 2012). A similar approach that takes issues of power and equity into account was promoted in Canada. A team of researchers worked with the citizens of the twin cities of Kitchener-Waterloo to promote community integration for people with long-term mental health problems. This project identified some key factors for success: stakeholder participation and empowerment, community support and integration, social justice and access to valued resources. Each factor was necessary to promote inclusion and challenge exclusion and required community workers to work with individuals and groups in the community (Nelson *et al.* 2001).

Community development approaches can help to tackle social exclusion for mental health service users and help promote a wider sense of mental well-being for community members (Morris and Gilchrist 2011; Schneider 2009). Community development works from the bottom up, not from the top down and so requires skills in connecting with people from diverse backgrounds. The role of a community development worker is quite different to that of most mental health professionals, being less boundaried and more wide ranging. Unfortunately, funding for such work is dependent on the prevailing political climate, and community development workers do not enjoy the status accorded to other professionals (Seebohm, Gilchrist and Morris 2012). There are thus a number of challenges to establishing this type of role alongside those of the more traditional mental health workers found in most towns and cities.

Social support initiatives in the community

Whether or not a particular locality employs workers with a remit for promoting community integration, there are a number of organisations and groups that offer socially supportive services and activities in the community. This section looks at some of the types of initiatives that may be found in many parts of the UK and beyond and what sort of support they are likely to offer.

Supported living

At the most basic level, people need somewhere to live that meets their requirements for physical comfort and psychological security. For many people, these needs may be met in their own homes, but some people, either because of isolation or having high levels of support needs, can benefit from living in supported housing. Following the closure of the old, long-stay hospital wards, housing schemes with varying levels of support have been set up, often in collaboration with housing associations or third-sector mental health organisations. At the most supportive end are hostels with onsite staff available around the clock. At the other end are group homes that just receive occasional visits from a support worker. These types of accommodation can provide supportive social networks for service users, although they do not seem to encourage the development of social networks unconnected with mental health (Dayson *et al.* 1998; Forrester-Jones *et al.* 2012).

Daytime occupation

For the many service users who are not in employment, there is still a need for something to do in the day and for social contact with other people. Since the deinstitutionalisation measures from the 1980s onwards, day centres have been created in many cities and some towns in the UK. Often run by third-sector organisations such as Mind and the Richmond Fellowship, they can be either a drop-in facility or one for which formal referral is required. In the past, it was sufficient to offer somewhere to be, have coffee and lunch and perhaps engage in some recreational or creative activities. Increasingly, the local authority funders are requiring a more formal approach in which service users are supported towards various self-development goals. This inevitably changes the nature of the experience and leads to the provision of more structured activities. As day centres take on new identities such as 'well-being centres' to meet these demands, it may become increasingly rare to encounter a purely recreational service for adults of working age.

Clubhouses (also mentioned in Chapter 6), which originated in the USA, offer a slightly different model for daytime occupation in which there is a blend of social, educational and employment-based activities. Clubhouses are run by members and may operate as social enterprises. In the USA, they have been associated with transitional employment schemes in which the clubhouse undertakes that a mainstream job will be fulfilled but with flexibility around who actually does that job on any one day. Clubhouse members report high levels of satisfaction with the social support they receive as a result of their involvement (Carolan *et al.* 2011). There are only a few mental health clubhouses in the UK at present but they offer a useful model of a resource that can meet a range of needs for service users, from providing somewhere to be to finding employment.

A diversity of organisations across the UK act as resource centres, mental health hubs and centres for a range of advisory, educational, recreational, creative and therapeutic activities. One example is the Falkirk and District Association for Mental Health in Scotland that offers a wide range of opportunities including: befriending, drop-in, counselling, support in linking to other services and activity groups and support groups as well as help and information services (Falkirk and District Association for Mental Health 2014). A centre such as this can act as a one-stop shop for a range of needs and can enable progression between activities in a way that avoids difficult transitions between groups or services.

Peer support: self-help groups

As has been mentioned previously, service users often value advice and support from others who have been through similar experiences to themselves. Peer support can take place on a one-to-one basis in person or on the telephone, as part of an activity-focused group (for example knitting or walking) or as part of an organised befriending programme (Temperley *et al.* 2013). Peer support in groups often has a self-help focus and these groups may or may not be facilitated. Where facilitation occurs, this may be provided by a peer supporter or by a mental health professional.

Peer support and self-help groups can be found in the types of organisations mentioned above and they can also be freestanding and independent, meeting in hired premises or operating largely online. Some self-help groups are generic, whereas others have a particular focus such as: depression, bipolar experiences, hearing voices, sexual abuse, alcohol addiction, etc. (Basset *et al.* 2010). Whatever the initial focus, the purpose of these groups seems to include improving mental well-being, becoming empowered, sharing coping strategies, obtaining emotional support and increasing resilience (Seebohm *et al.* 2013). A common feature of self-help groups seems to be the development of trust, which creates a safe space in which to talk about issues that would be difficult to address in other social situations. Another type of group, focusing on service user/survivor issues, tends to be explicitly involved in campaigning, emancipatory action and civil rights activities (Campbell 2009).

Befriending schemes

Some individuals can become very isolated as a result of their mental distress and the thought of participating in social situations can be extremely anxiety-provoking. This is where befriending schemes can help. Isolated individuals are matched with a volunteer, often drawn from the same locality, who will meet up with them on a regular basis and encourage them to be out and about in the community. Volunteers are trained to maintain appropriate boundaries and are provided with supervision so that any safety concerns can be picked up. The relationship has elements of a typical friendship, as it is based on having time to talk and enjoying doing activities together. However, organised befriending places tighter boundaries around the relationship than would be the case for a naturally occurring friendship and there is less expectation of reciprocity. Despite being more formalised than other types of friendship, befriending partnerships are valued by service users and there is some emerging evidence of their contribution to improving mental well-being (McGowan and Jowett 2003; Mead *et al.* 2010; Temperley *et al.* 2013).

Community activities

The activities mentioned so far in this section are ones specifically developed for people with mental health problems. For some people who are feeling particularly vulnerable, these settings, where their difficulties will be taken into account, may be all that they feel they can manage. By contrast, some may prefer not to use mental health facilities at all, choosing to engage directly in mainstream community activities. For others, a mix of the two may best meet their needs; mental-health-specific contexts for support and understanding, community activities to meet a wider range of people and to feel part of 'normal life'.

As for anyone in the community with time on their hands, there are a range of activities that can provide meaningful occupation and companionship. Most towns and cities will have lists of faith groups, clubs and societies, volunteering opportunities and community education classes that can be joined. In some locations, there are 'time banks', where people can offer to help others in a range of ways and in return can receive help themselves without having to do a direct swap (Simon 2010). 'Local exchange trading schemes' or 'LETS' are another example of a way of connecting with people locally. Unlike time banks, LETS allow goods as well as services to be traded and, rather than keeping an account of hours spent, local tokens are used to value the exchanges (Aldridge *et al.* 2001). Such schemes can be valuable in community development and in having access to low-cost practical assistance.

For older people, connecting to community can be important for health and well-being. There have been a number of recent initiatives attempting to address issues of isolation amongst the increasing numbers of older people in society (Bartley 2012). Older people can have particular issues of loneliness and isolation arising from becoming less mobile and through the loss of friends, partners and other relatives over time (Allan 1989). Age UK, local authorities and other organisations provide lunch clubs, yoga classes, day centres and other activities for older citizens. The University of the Third Age offers opportunities to get together and learn about a whole range of subjects. There is a growing body of research about the social and other needs of older people (Joseph Rowntree Foundation 2013). This is an area that is likely to see a growth in interest as the implications of a steadily ageing population are recognised.

Conclusion: the challenges for social support

Health and social care policy has started to embrace the importance of the broader social context in service users' lives. Personalisation offers opportunities to engage with a wider range of activities that can improve well-being. If these policies genuinely translate into opportunities for service users to use personal budgets for self-directed support then they may choose to engage in activities that fall outside of traditional service provision. Practitioners will need to find new, more flexible ways of working and service users will need information and, in some cases, assistance to make informed choices about their support options. If social support options are to compete with, or complement, medical and psychological services on the road to recovery, the benefits of and the rationale for this approach will need to be clearly set out.

This chapter has looked at a number of ways that service users can become more connected with social networks and thus engage in giving and receiving social support. Staff, volunteers and fellow participants in these different projects could all enhance the social support they provide by considering the nature of that support and the elements of it that work best in their particular context. Chapter 4 described five categories of social support: engaging in friendship, providing emotional support, constructing meaning, offering practical advice and giving material assistance. Each of these is likely to be present to some extent in every context, but depending on the nature of the setting, some will be more to the fore than others. Although the informality of that support is one of its strengths, there could still be benefits in offering training sessions that highlight the most effective ways of enabling that support and discuss the boundaries within which social supporters need to operate.

Chapter 9

Conclusion

Introduction

Social support seems to be fundamental to human life; most of our basic and higher needs can only be met through the give and take of collaboration with other people. Evolutionary theorists suggest that our brains are larger than those of other animals because of the need to communicate with others in the complex ways that enable highly developed social organisation and the maintenance of personal relationships (Dunbar 2010). Our very survival as a species has been dependent on our ability to communicate and cooperate with other human beings. So the suggestion that social support should be available to people affected by mental health problems is not to offer charity, but rather to extend the opportunities that most of the population benefit from in their daily lives. In this way, social support fits very well with approaches to mental health that focus on facilitating recovery and tackling social exclusion (Repper and Perkins 2003; Tew 2013).

The importance of social support

It is notable that psychological therapies and many other treatments do not set out to help mentally distressed people cope with lives of social isolation; rather they look at how the relationship between self and others can be a healthy and satisfying one. So it seems only logical to view mental health as having both personal and social elements. Unfortunately, the personal and individualised perspectives on mental health, as seen in bio-medical and psychological approaches, have tended to overshadow the social perspective. Look in any academic bookshop and there will be rows of books on psychiatry, psychotherapy and counselling, but you will be hard pressed to find more than a handful of volumes on a social approach to mental health. Sociologists have long been interested in the impact of the social world on mental health and distress, but on the whole this has been an academic interest rather than one that has sought to come up with practical solutions to the problems being studied. One notable exception to this is found in the work of George Brown and Tirril Harris who tested befriending interventions with depressed women (Brown *et al.* 1986; Harris *et al.* 1999).

Generally, sociologists have tended to take a critical stance in questioning the concept of mental illness and the role of psychiatrists. Although there are good reasons for being critical, this tendency may have been partly responsible for the downplaying of the value of a sociological understanding and its implications by practitioners in the mental health field (Pilgrim and Rogers 2005). Another barrier may be that a number of sociological writers tend to present their ideas in a rather rarefied and inaccessible style that is off-putting to readers who have not had the benefit of studying social sciences at degree level. This way of presenting sociological ideas may be a reaction to fears that the discipline, as it reports on social phenomena, may be seen as more like journalism than science unless it is presented using complex language. When sociological ideas can be communicated more clearly, they stand a better chance of informing the actions of those who want to bring about social change, such as by challenging the exclusion and discrimination faced by people with mental health problems.

In contrast to psychiatry, nursing or applied psychology, where practitioners have a certain level of status and power, the domain of social support is more informal and intuitive in its approach. People working in this field tend not to have the same trappings of professional status, for instance membership of a professional regulating body, career structures and grades and training that covers defined areas of knowledge and skills. Although the social work profession in mental health encompasses a social support element, it is more formally structured and dependent on the relationship with psychiatry than those approaches that are mainly informed by social perspectives (Tew *et al.* 2012). The lack of both status and perceived professionalism associated with social support roles present a dilemma in the mental health field. The very informality makes such support accessible to service users and is a relatively low-cost option, however it does not receive the recognition it deserves and so there is considerable variation in the availability and quality of social support across the UK and other countries. As much social support comes from family, friends, neighbours and colleagues, much of it sits outside the realm of professional practice anyway.

A social understanding of mental health

This book has attempted to demonstrate that ideas developed in the fields of sociology, social anthropology and social-psychology can have practical relevance for the empowerment of people who have been disadvantaged as a result of having experienced mental health problems. Although such problems do have troubling personal impacts on thoughts, feelings, motivation and behaviour at times, there are also significant external barriers to recovery and participation in society that require a social perspective on the situation. There are many parallels with the social model of disability, first developed by people with physical and sensory impairments, which points to the disabling effects of a society that fails to accommodate the diverse needs of those who do not match an idealised healthy norm (Beresford 2009). Whatever role biological or psychological traits may or may not play, social factors such as inequalities, unemployment, poverty, poor housing, domestic violence, sexual abuse and discrimination are recognised as risk factors in triggering and maintaining mental distress (Tew *et al.* 2012; U'ren 2011).

Social forces play a key role in defining what is accepted as reality and often attempt to control and constrain those who do not share the dominant view of how the world is constructed (Berger and Luckman 1967). Someone who is very depressed or hears voices could be seen as deviating from the dominant culture's reality and thus to occupy the position of an outsider. Similarly, personal identity is shaped through interactions with others and certain identities are devalued or stigmatised, often because certain groups in society are labelled and stereotyped rather than being viewed as sharing a common humanity (Jenkins 2008; Link and Phelan 2010). Service users may find themselves expected to occupy a 'sick role' (Parsons 1951) and while that may offer some short-term benefits, in the longer term it can become disempowering. In response to these negative social forces, service user and survivor movements have sought to promote a more positive identity and to argue for a greater tolerance of diversity within society (Campbell 2009).

Social support, especially at the informal end, is closely linked to the notion of friendship. Although making friends is a very personal affair, there are some quite well-established social patterns that influence whether or not people are likely to become friends and if that friendship is likely to last. Individuals tend to have friends who occupy a similar status to themselves. Friendships that are not reciprocal in the attention and support given to each other over the long term are not likely to persist (Allan 1989). Most people only seem to be able maintain a small number of close friendships at any one time, although there can be many others with whom there is occasional contact (Dunbar 2010). Only one or two people within a friendship network may be confided in about personal health issues, but their views can be quite influential in the process of deciding how to address those issues (Perry and Pescosolido 2010).

The support that is exchanged with family, friends and others can help to affirm a positive identity and act as a buffer against the stresses and strains encountered in life. Research into the nature of social support shows that the same elements are offered and valued both in the general population and amongst those who have been diagnosed as having mental health conditions (Burleson, Albrecht and Sarason 1994; Faulkner and Layzell 2000; Milne 1999). As mentioned throughout this book, those elements of social support can be divided into five categories: friendship, emotional support, finding meaning, offering advice and providing material assistance. It is not necessary for all these five elements to be offered by any one person, and each individual will vary in what type of support they feel they need. Nor are the five categories rigidly separated. It would be quite possible, for example, to offer practical assistance to help someone to manage their financial affairs in an emotionally supportive manner.

The five elements should not be regarded as a social prescription to be dispensed without consideration of each person's situation or without paying attention to the potential pitfalls associated with some of those elements. In Chapter 4, the giving of advice was identified as a complex area, as it may not be welcome or be appropriate to the recipient's circumstances. Material assistance can relieve practical problems, but some people can feel embarrassed about being seen as needy and having a sense of indebtedness to others. Emotional support tends to be highly valued but raises some issues for consideration. The opening up of strong emotions or 'catharsis' is not particularly difficult to achieve, but the results can be unpredictable and uncomfortable for the parties involved; not everyone is well equipped to deal with the outpouring of powerful emotions. A relationship in which emotional issues are frequently aired may risk giving too much attention to the negative aspects of life and may re-stimulate rather than deal with distress. Another risk is that sustained emotional intensity around difficult issues can cause the person in the supporting role to suffer 'burnout' and feel unable to sustain the relationship. None of this is to deny the benefits of an empathetic relationship, but rather to ask for some awareness of how far it is appropriate to go when offering support.

The building of positive and empowering relationships needs to be based on clear foundations including: mutual respect, trust, being non-judgemental and a belief that both parties have something to bring to the relationship. The more equal is the status of the two people in a social relationship, the more likely it is to feel as if it is a friendship. For mental health practitioners, there are professional boundaries and power imbalances, which mean that, although they can operate in a friendly manner, they cannot truly be 'friends' with the users of their services. For social supporters, the situation is less clear. At the informal end of the spectrum, much social support is provided by friends and family where the relationship is based on mutual liking or a sense of kinship obligation. At the more formal end, staff working in third-sector community projects, employment support schemes, social enterprises, etc. are likely to have a more relaxed relationship with service users than would apply in a clinical setting but still with certain boundaries in place. In the middle ground, are people in roles such as peer supporters and volunteer befrienders who offer much of the support associated with friendship but are doing so in a more structured way.

Promoting social support
Social support for people with mental health problems can be broadly divided into two types. First, there is the support that flows from having

friends, family and regular contact with people in the community, workplace or other setting. Second, there is the organised form of support provided by drop-in centres, clubhouses, self-help groups and the like, which intentionally set out to sustain everyday living. Ideally, the latter type of support would aim to connect the people who use it with the informal level of support found in social networks so that they are involved in mainstream, rather than segregated, social interactions.

Organisations that support mental health service users in the community could benefit from exploring the practical implication of the concepts of social networks and social capital in relation to their own localities. What form does social capital take in their area and what connections do they have that could enable service users to benefit from that capital? Are there opportunities for both bonding capital, where people in the same situation can collaborate with each other for mutual support, and bridging capital, where new opportunities for work and leisure are opened up by making connections across different groups? So, for instance, this might involve setting up service user self-help groups on the one hand and liaising with potential employers on the other hand. These community-based organisations could take time to find out about the social networks of their users and work with them to help them extend these networks or even to find additional ones to join.

Mainstream mental health services and service commissioners could look at supporting the work of community-based organisations that help service users connect to networks of natural support. Although some financial investment would be required, there is likely to be a payback in terms of the improved quality of life of service users, an increase in informal support and most likely a reduced need for use of clinical services (Samuel 2013). The employment of community development workers could be considered, as they can work at a grass-roots level in communities, facilitating networks and supporting individuals to become more connected (Seebohm et al. 2012). Mental health services could also make greater use of a 'Support Time and Recovery' worker whose role has been specifically developed to support service users to live independently in the community. The introduction of personal health and social care budgets for self-directed support offers an opportunity for case managers working in services to help users access social networks in their community.

Outside of service provision, service user/survivor and self-help organisations show that support initiatives can come from the bottom up, often in very creative ways that are less likely to have occurred within mainstream services. Examples of this include hearing-voices groups, crisis telephone support lines, crisis support houses, anti-stigma campaigns, holistic and alternative therapies, use of theatre, poetry, creative writing and art as well as training and research groups (Stastny and Lehman 2007; Wallcraft 2009). In educational and employment settings, social support can play a key role in helping to gain employment and to maintain a job or to achieve a qualification. Most people in these contexts use social support to help them through difficult situations and that support especially needs to be available to those who are feeling more vulnerable.

Another way of promoting social support is through research, education and training. Social aspects of mental health tend not to attract the levels of funding received for the evaluation of bio-medical or psychological interventions. Nevertheless, there is a steady stream of research articles and reports that explore what service users want in their lives and that evaluate the contribution social approaches are making to meeting their needs. The Social Perspectives Network (Social Perspectives Network 2014), founded in 2002, brings together social workers, academics, service users and others interested in this approach and shares information on research and training matters. At the time of writing, the Royal Society for the Arts is over halfway through a major research project in England testing and evaluating interventions designed to improve mental well-being through strengthening social networks (Morris and Gilchrist 2011). The Institute of Mental Health based at The University of Nottingham has just launched a new Centre for Social Futures to work with service users, carers and professionals to advance understanding of social and cultural interventions for mental health recovery and to help to address inequalities associated with having mental health problems (SoFu 2014). In many ways, there has never been a better time to promote the value of social support for mental health.

Final words

In emphasising the importance of informal social support in the community, there is a risk of inadvertently sanctioning withdrawal of funding from mainstream health and social care services. Ever since government policy has moved away from long-stay treatment in mental hospitals, there have been concerns that many service users have been let down by a lack of adequate alternatives in the name of 'community care'. At a time when mental health services are struggling to meet the demands made upon them with limited resources, there is a danger of different sectors feeling that they are competing with each other. Given the huge social and economic costs of mental health problems to society, it could be argued that all the different sectors involved in providing treatment and support should press for greater levels of funding. Psychiatry has many critics, some of them psychiatrists themselves, and there is still a debate to be had about the strengths and weaknesses of bio-medical, psychological and social approaches for resolving mental health problems. Whatever the outcomes of those debates (based on evidence, it is hoped), it would seem that there is a role for social support as an important element in both reducing the risk of developing a mental health problem and in promoting recovery. If this book and others like it can raise awareness of the importance of the social world that service users and others affected by mental health issues inhabit, then there is a chance that social support will be taken more seriously.

References

Addington, J., van Mastrigt, S., Hutchinson, J. and Addington, D. (2002) 'Pathways to care: help seeking behaviour in first episode psychosis.' *Acta Psychiatrica Scandinavica 106*, 358–364.

Albrecht, T. and Adelman, M. (1987) *Communicating Social Support.* Thousand Oaks: Sage.

Aldridge, T., Tooke, J., Lee, R., Leyshon, A., Thrift, N. and Williams, C. (2001) 'Recasting work: the example of local exchange trading schemes.' *Work, Employment and Society 15,* 3, 565–579.

Alekeson, V. and Rumbold, B. (2013) *Personal Health Budgets: Challengers for Commissioners and Policy-Makers.* London: Nuffield Trust. Available at www.nuffieldtrust.org.uk/ sites/files/nuffield/publication/130828_personal_health_budgets_summary. pdf, accessed on 24 July 2014.

Alexander, J. (2001) 'Depressed men: an exploratory study of close relationships.' *Journal of Psychiatric and Mental Health Nursing 8,* 1, 67–75.

Allan, G. (1989) *Friendship.* Hemel Hempstead: Harvester Wheatsheaf.

Allan, G. (1996) *Kinship and Friendship in Modern Britain.* Oxford: Oxford University Press.

Allan, G. (2001) 'Personal relationships in late modernity.' *Personal Relationships 8,* 325–339.

Allan, G. (2008) 'Flexibility, friendship, and family.' *Personal Relationships 15,* 1–16.

Allan, G. (2011) 'Commentary: friendships and emotions.' *Sociological Research Online 16,* 1, 15. Available at www.socresonline.org.uk/16/1/15.html, accessed on 24 July 2014.

Andrews, B. and Wilding, J. (2004) 'The relation of depression and anxiety to life-stress and achievement in students.' *British Journal of Psychology 95,* 509–521.

Apter, T. (2001) *The Myth of Maturity: What Teenagers Need from Parents to Become Adults.* New York: W.W. Norton and Company.

Argyle, M. (1991) *Cooperation: The Basis of Sociability.* London: Routledge.

Argyle, M., Bryant, B. and Trower, P. (1974) 'Social skills training and psychotherapy: a comparative study.' *Psychological Medicine 4,* 435–443.

Askey, R., Holmshaw, J. Gamble, C. and Gray, R. (2009) 'What do carers of people with psychosis need from mental health services? Exploring the views of carers, service users and professionals.' *Journal of Family Therapy 31,* 310–331.

Bagley, C. (2011) 'From Sure Start to Children's Centres: capturing the erosion of social capital.' *Journal of Educational Policy 26*, 1, 95–113.

Barker, C., and Pistrang, N. (2002) 'Psychotherapy and social support: integrating research on psychological helping.' *Clinical Psychology Review 22*, 3, 361–379.

Barnard, K. and Lloyd, C. (2012) 'Experiencing Depression and Diabetes.' In C. Lloyd and T. Heller (eds) *Long-Term Conditions: Challenges in Health and Social Care.* London: Sage.

Barnes, M. and Duck, M. (1994) 'Everyday Communicative Contexts for Social Support.' In B. Burleson, T. Albrecht and I. Sarason (eds) *Communication of Social Support: Messages, Interactions, Relationships and Community.* Thousand Oaks: Sage.

Bartley, M. (ed.) (2012) *Life Gets Under Your Skin.* London: UCL Research Department of Epidemiology and Public Health. Available at www.ucl.ac.uk/icls/publications/booklets/lguys.pdf, accessed on 24 July 2014.

Basset, T., Faulkner, A., Repper, J. and Stamou, E. (2010) *Lived Experience Leading the Way: Peer Support in Mental Health.* London: Together. Available at www.nsun.org.uk/assets/downloadableFiles/livedexperiencereport.pdf, accessed on 24 July 2014.

Bassett, E. and Moore, S. (2013) *Mental Health and Social Capital: Social Capital as a Promising Initiative to Improving the Mental Health of Communities.* Rijeka: InTech. Available at http://dx.doi.org/10.5772/53501, accessed on 24 July 2014.

Basu, K. (2010) 'The moral basis of prosperity and oppression: altruism, other-regarding behavior and identity.' *Economics and Philosophy 26*, 189–216.

Batson, C. (2010) 'The naked emperor: seeking a more plausible genetic basis for psychological altruism.' *Economics and Philosophy 26*, 149–164.

Beavan, V., Read, J. and Cartwright, C. (2011) 'The prevalence of voice-hearers in the general population: a literature review.' *Journal of Mental Health 20*, 3, 281–292.

Bentall, R. (2004) *Madness Explained: Psychosis and Human Nature.* London: Penguin.

Bentall, R. (2010) *Doctoring the Mind: Why Psychiatric Treatments Fail.* London: Penguin.

Beresford, P. (2009) 'Thinking about "Mental Health": Towards a Social Model.' In J. Reynolds, R. Muston, T. Heller, J. Leach, M. McCormick, J. Wallcraft and M. Walsh (eds) *Mental Health Still Matters.* Basingstoke: Palgrave Macmillan.

Berger, P. and Luckman, T. (1967) *The Social Construction of Reality.* Harmondsworth: Penguin.

Berne, E. (1964) *Games People Play: The Psychology of Human Relationships.* London: Penguin.

Bewick, B., Koutsopoulou, G., Miles, J., Slaa, E. and Barkham, M. (2010) 'Changes in undergraduate students' psychological well-being as they progress through university.' *Studies in Higher Education 35*, 6, 633–645.

Bolger, N. and Amarel, D. (2007) 'Effects of social support visibility on adjustment to stress; experimental evidence.' *Journal of Personality and Social Psychology 92*, 3, 458–475.

Bolton, D. (2010) 'Conceptualisation of mental disorder and its personal meanings.' *Journal of Mental Health 19*, 4, 328–336.

Borg, M. and Davidson, L. (2008) 'The nature of recovery as lived in everyday experience.' *Journal of Mental Health 17,* 2, 129–140.

Borthwick, A., Holam, C., Kennard, D., McFetridge, M., Messruther, K. and Wilkes, J. (2001) 'The relevance of moral treatment to contemporary mental health care.' *Journal of Mental Health 10,* 4, 427–439.

Bostock, J., Kitt, R. and Kitt, C. (2011) 'Why wait until qualified?: the benefits and experiences of undergoing mental health awareness training for PGCE students.' *Pastoral Care in Education 29,* 2, 103–115.

Bourdieu, P. (1986) 'The Forms of Capital.' In J. Richardson (ed.) *Handbook of Theory and Research for the Sociology of Education.* New York: Greenwood Press.

Bouteyre, E., Maurel, M. and Bernaud, J.L. (2007) 'Daily hassles and depressive symptoms among first year psychology students in France: the role of coping and social support.' *Stress and Health 23,* 93–99.

Brackett, M., Rivers, S. and Salovey, P. (2011) 'Emotional intelligence: implications for personal, social, academic, and workplace success.' *Social and Personality Psychology Compass 5,* 1, 88–103.

Bradshaw, W., Armour, M.P. and Roseborough, D. (2007) 'Finding a place in the world: the experience of recovery from severe mental illness.' *Qualitative Social Work 6,* 1, 27–47.

Bridgett, C. and Polak, P. (2003) 'Social systems intervention and crisis resolution. Part 1: assessment.' *Advances in Psychiatric Treatment 9,* 6, 424–431.

Brindle, D. (2012) 'Welsh government unveils social care reform plans.' *The Guardian,* 13 March. Available at www.theguardian.com/social-care-network/2012/mar/13/welsh-government-social-care-reform, accessed on 24 July 2014.

Brindle, D. (2013) 'Remploy factories shut up shop – the end of an era for disabled workers.' *The Guardian,* 30 October. Available at www.theguardian.com/society/2013/oct/30/remploy-factories-close-disabled-workers, accessed on 24 July 2014.

Brown, G., Andrews, B., Harris, T., Adler, Z. and Bridge, L. (1986) 'Social support, self-esteem and depression.' *Psychological Medicine 16,* 813–831.

Browne, D. (2009) 'Black Communities, Mental Health and the Criminal Justice System.' In J. Reynolds, R. Muston, T. Heller, J. Leach, M. McCormick, J. Wallcraft and M. Walsh (eds) *Mental Health Still Matters.* Basingstoke: Palgrave Macmillan.

Burleson, B., Albrecht, T. and Sarason, I. (eds) (1994) *Communication of Social Support: Messages, Interactions, Relationships and Community.* Thousand Oaks: Sage.

Burleson, B. (1994) 'Comforting Messages: Significance, Approaches and Effects.' In B. Burleson, T. Albrecht and I. Sarason (eds) *Communication of Social Support: Messages, Interactions, Relationships and Community.* Thousand Oaks: Sage.

Burns, T. (2006) *Psychiatry: A Very Short Introduction.* Oxford: Oxford University Press.

Burns, T., Catty, J., Becker, T., Drake, R. *et al.* (2007) 'The effectiveness of supported employment for people with severe mental illness: a randomised controlled trial.' *The Lancet 370,* 1146–1152.

Burton, D. and Goodman, R. (2011) 'Perspectives of SENcos and support staff in England on their roles and capacity to support inclusive practice for students with behavioural emotional and social difficulties.' *Pastoral Care in Education 29*, 2, 133–149.

Butterworth, P., Leach, L., Strazdins, L., Oleson, S., Rodgers, B. and Broom, D. (2011) 'The psychosocial quality of work determines whether employment has benefits for mental health: results from a longitudinal national household panel survey.' *Occupational and Environmental Medicine 68*, 806–812.

Buzlaff, R. and Hooley, J. (1998) 'Expressed emotion and psychiatric relapse.' *Archives of General Psychiatry 55*, 547–552.

Cable, N., Bartley, M., Chandola, T. and Sacker, A. (2013) 'Friends are equally important to men and women, but family matters more for men's well-being.' *Journal of Epidemiology and Community Health 67,* 2, 166–171.

Cacioppo, J. and Cacioppo, S. (2014) 'Social relationships and health: the toxic effects of perceived social isolation.' *Social and Personality Psychology Compass 8*, 2, 58–72.

Cacioppo, J., Hawkley, T. and Thisted, R. (2010) 'Perceived isolation makes me sad.' *Psychology of Aging 25*, 453–463.

Cain, S. (2012) *Quiet: the Power of Introverts in a World That Can't Stop Talking.* London: Penguin.

Cameron, J., Walker, C., Hart, A., Sadlo, G. and Haslam, I. (2012) 'Supporting workers with mental health problems to retain employment: users' experiences of a UK job retention project.' *Work: A Journal of Prevention, Assessment and Rehabilitation 42*, 4, 461–471.

Campbell, P. (2009) 'The Service User/Survivor Movement.' In J. Reynolds, R. Muston, T. Heller, J. Leach, M. McCormick, J. Wallcraft and M. Walsh (eds) *Mental Health Still Matters.* Basingstoke: Palgrave Macmillan.

Cantó-Milà, N. and Seebach, S. (2011) 'Ana's friends: friendship in online pro-ana communities.' *Sociological Research Online 16*, 1. Available at www.socresonline. org.uk/16/1/1.html, accessed on 24 July 2014.

Carolan, M., Onaga, E., Pernice-Duca, F. and Jimenez, T. (2011) 'A place to be: the role of Clubhouses in facilitating social support.' *Psychiatric Rehabilitation Journal 35,* 2, 125–132.

Carpenter, M. and Raj, T. (2012) 'Editorial introduction: towards a paradigm shift from community care to community development in mental health.' *Community Development Journal 47*, 4, 457–472.

Carr, A. (2006) *Family Therapy: Concepts, Process and Practice.* Chichester: Wiley.

Centre for Independent Living NI (2011) *Personalisation, Self-Directed Support and Personal Budgets.* Belfast: Centre for Independent Living NI. Available at www. cilbelfast.org/content/personalisation-self-directed-support-and-personal-budgets-0, accessed on 24 July 2014.

Chaney, D. (2002) *Cultural Change and Everyday Life.* Basingstoke: Palgrave.

Chao, R. (2011) 'Managing stress and maintaining well-being: social support, problem-focused coping and avoidant coping.' *Journal of Counseling and Development 89*, 338–348.

Chappell, N. and Funk, L (2010) 'Social capital: does it add to the health inequalities debate?' *Social Indicators Research 99*, 3, 357–373.

Chew-Graham, C., Rogers, A. and Yassim, N. (2003) '"I wouldn't want it on my CV or their records": medical students' experience of help-seeking for mental health problems.' *Medical Education 37*, 873–880.

Ciarrochi, J. and Deane, F. (2001) 'Emotional competence and willingness to seek help from professional and non-professional sources.' *British Journal of Counselling and Guidance 29*, 2, 233–246.

Clatworthy, J., Hinds, J. and Camic, P. (2013) 'Gardening as a mental health intervention: a review.' *Mental Health Review Journal 18*, 4, 214–225.

Clift, S. and Morrison, I. (2011) 'Group singing fosters mental health and wellbeing: findings from the East Kent "singing for health" network project.' *Mental Health and Social Inclusion 15*, 2, 88–97.

Colombo, A., Bendelow, G., Fulford, B. and Williams S. (2003) 'Evaluating the influence of implicit models of mental disorder on processes of shared decision making within community-based multi-disciplinary teams.' *Social Science and Medicine 56*, 1557–1570.

Community Care (2013) 'The state of personalisation 2013.' *Community Care.* Available at www.communitycare.co.uk/state-of-personalisation-2013/#.UrIZ8PRdWHh, accessed on 24 July 2014.

Cook, K. and Whitmeyer, J. (1992). 'Two approaches to social structure: exchange theory and network analysis.' *Annual Review of Sociology 1992*, 109–127.

Cooper, P. (2011a) 'Teacher strategies for effective intervention with students presenting social, emotional and behavioural difficulties: an international review.' *European Journal of Special Needs Education 26*, 1, 71–86.

Cooper, P. (2011b) 'Teacher strategies for effective intervention with students presenting social, emotional and behavioural difficulties: implications for policy and practice.' *European Journal of Special Needs Education 26*, 1, 87–92.

Cornford, C., Hill, A. and Reilly, J. (2007) 'How patients with depressive symptoms view their condition: a qualitative study.' *Family Practice 24*, 358–364.

Corry, P. (2008) *Stigma Shout: Service User and Carer Experiences of Stigma and Discrimination.* London: Time to Change.

Craig, T. (2008) 'Recovery: say what you mean and mean what you say.' *Journal of Mental Health 17*, 2, 125–128.

Crawford, P., Lewis, L., Brown, B. and Manning, N. (2013) 'Creative practice as mutual recovery in mental health.' *Mental Health Review Journal 18*, 2, 55–64.

Dayson, D., Lee-Jones, R., Chahal, K. and Leff, J. (1998) 'The TAPS Project 32: social networks of two group homes… 5 years on.' *Social Psychiatry and Psychiatric Epidemiology 33*, 9, 438–444.

De Silva, M., McKenzie, K., Harpham, T. and Huttly, S. (2005) 'Social capital and mental illness: a systematic review.' *Journal of Epidemiology and Community Health 59*, 8, 619–627.

Deegan, P. (1988) 'Recovery: the lived experience of rehabilitation.' *Psychosocial Rehabilitation Journal 11*, 11–19.

Department for Work and Pensions (2009) *Realising Ambitions: Better Employment Support for People with a Mental Health Condition.* London: The Stationery Office.

Department of Health (2010) *Recognised, Valued and Supported: Next Steps for the Carers Strategy.* London: Department of Health.

Department of Health (2011) *No Health Without Mental Health.* London: Department of Health.

Department of Health (2012) *IAPT Three-year Report: the First Million Patients.* London: Department of Health.

Department of Health (2014) *Closing the Gap: Priorities for Essential Change in Mental Health.* London: Department of Health.

Dunbar, R. (2010) *How Many Friends Does One Person Need? Dunbar's Number and Other Evolutionary Quirks.* London: Faber and Faber.

Durkheim, E. (1971) 'Anomic Suicide.' In K. Thompson and J. Tunstall (eds) *Sociological Perspectives.* Harmondsworth: Penguin.

Earwaker, J. (1992) *Helping and Supporting Students: Re-thinking the Issues.* Buckingham: Society for Research into Higher Education and The Open University.

Economic and Social Research Council (2013) *Evidence Briefing: Mental Health and Social Relationships.* London: Economic and Social Research Council. Available at www.esrc.ac.uk/_images/ESRC_Evidence_Briefing_Mental_health_social_rel_tcm8-26243.pdf, accessed on 24 July 2014.

Eisenberger, N., Jarcho, J., Lieberman, M. and Naliboff, B. (2006) 'An experimental study of shared sensitivity to physical pain and social rejection.' *Pain 126*, 1, 132–138.

El Ansari, W., Stock, C., Snelgrove, S., Hu, X. *et al.* (2011) 'Feeling healthy? A survey of physical and psychological wellbeing of students from seven universities in the UK.' *International Journal of Environmental Research and Public Health 8*, 5, 1308–1323.

Falkirk and District Association for Mental Health in Scotland (2014) *Falkirk's Association for Mental Health website.* Falkirk: Falkirk and District Association for Mental Health in Scotland. Available at www.fdamh.org.uk, accessed on 24 July 2014.

Farrand, P., Parker, M. and Lee, C. (2007) 'Intention of adolescents to seek professional help for emotional and behavioural difficulties.' *Health and Social Care in the Community 15*, 5, 464–473.

Faulkner, A. and Layzell, S. (2000) *Strategies for Living.* London: Mental Health Foundation.

Fernando, S. (2002) *Mental Health, Race and Culture.* Basingstoke: Palgrave.

Fetter, F.A. (1900) 'Recent discussion of the capital concept.' *The Quarterly Journal of Economics 15*, 1, 1–45.

Fieldhouse, J. (2012) 'Mental health, social inclusion, and community development: lessons from Bristol.' *Community Development Journal 47*, 4, 571–587.

Fisher, S. (1994) *Stress in Academic Life: The Mental Assembly Line.* Buckingham: Open University Press.

Forder, J., Jones, K., Glendinning, C., Caiels, J. *et al.* (2012) *Evaluation of the Personal Health Budget Pilot Programme, Discussion Paper, 2840-2.* Canterbury: PSSRU, University of Kent.

Forrester-Jones, R., Carpenter, J., Coolen-Schrijner, P., Cambridge, P., Tate, A., Hallam, A. and Wooff, D. (2012) 'Good friends are hard to find? The social networks of people with mental illness 12 years after deinstitutionalisation.' *Journal of Mental Health 21,* 1, 4–14.

Foucault, M. (1965) *Madness and Civilization: A History of Insanity in the Age of Reason.* New York: Random House.

Fox, K. (2004) *Watching the English: The Hidden Rules of English Behaviour.* London: Hodder and Stoughton.

Furedi, F. (2004) *Therapy Culture: Cultivating Vulnerability in an Uncertain Age.* London: Routledge.

Gelder, M., Mayou, R. and Geddes, J. (2005) *Psychiatry* (2nd edition). Oxford: Oxford University Press.

Geys, B. and Murdoch, Z. (2010) 'Measuring the "bridging" versus "bonding" nature of social networks: a proposal for integrating existing measures.' *Sociology 44,* 3, 523–540.

Gibney, A., Moore, N., Murphy, F. and O'Sullivan, S. (2011) 'The first semester of university life; "will I be able to manage it all?"' *Higher Education 62*, 3, 351–366.

Giddens, A. (1990) *The Consequences of Modernity.* London: Polity Press.

Gilbert, E., Marwaha, S., Milton, A., Johnson, S. *et al.* (2013) 'Social firms as a means of vocational recovery for people with mental illness: a UK survey' *BMC Health Services Research 13*, 1, 270.

Gilchrist, A. (2004) *The Well-Connected Community: A Networking Approach to Community Development.* Bristol: The Policy Press.

Giordano, G. and Lindström, M. (2011) 'Social capital and change in psychological health over time.' *Social Science and Medicine 72*, 8, 1219–1227.

Glasby, J. (2007) *Understanding Health and Social Care.* Bristol: The Policy Press.

Glendinning, C., Challis, D., Fernandez, J., Jacobs, S. *et al.* (2008) *Evaluation of the Individual Budgets Pilot Programme: Final Report.* York: Social Policy Research Unit, University of York. Available at www.york.ac.uk/inst/spru/pubs/pdf/IBSEN. pdf, accessed on 24 July 2014.

Goffman, E. (1961) *Asylums: Essays on the Social Situation of Mental Patients and Other Inmates.* New York: Doubleday.

Goffman, E. (1968) *Stigma: Notes on the Management of Spoiled Identity.* Harmondsworth: Pelican.

Goffman, E. (1971) *The Presentation of Self in Everyday Life.* Harmondsworth: Pelican.

Goldberg, D. and Huxley, P. (1992) *Common Mental Disorders: A Bio-social Model.* London: Routledge.

Goleman, D. (1996) *Emotional Intelligence: Why it Can Matter More Than IQ.* London: Bloomsbury.

Goleman, D. (1998) *Working with Emotional Intelligence.* London: Bloomsbury.

Grant, A. (2000) *Student Psychological Health Project.* Leicester: University of Leicester.

Green, G., Hayes, C., Dickinson, D., Whittaker, A. and Gilheany, B. (2002) 'The role and impact of social relationships upon well-being reported by mental health service users: a qualitative study.' *Journal of Mental Health 11*, 5, 565–579.

Green, H., McGinnity, A., Meltzer, H., Ford, T. and Goodman, R. (2005) *Mental Health of Children and Young People in Great Britain, 2004.* London: Office for National Statistics.

Grice, S., Kuipers, E., Bebbington, P., Dunn, G. *et al.* (2009) 'Carers' attributions about positive events in psychosis relate to expressed emotion.' *Behaviour Research and Therapy 47,* 9, 783–789.

Haddad, M., Walters, P. and Tylee, A. (2008) 'Mood disorders in primary care.' *Psychiatry 8*, 2, 71–75.

Halamandaris, K. (1995) *Correlates of Adjustment to University Life Among Students* (unpublished PhD thesis). Stirling: University of Stirling.

Halpern, D. (1995) *Mental Health and the Built Environment: More than Bricks and Mortar.* London: Taylor and Francis.

Hammond, C. (2004) 'Impacts of lifelong learning upon emotional resilience, psychological and mental health: fieldwork evidence.' *Oxford Review of Education 30*, 4, 551–568.

Hammond, J. (2012) 'Signpost: a model of self-directed support and a framework for brokerage.' *Mental Health and Social Inclusion 16*, 1, 48–55.

Hannigan, B. and Coffey, M. (2011) 'Where the wicked problems are: the case of mental health.' *Health Policy 101,* 3, 220–227.

Harris, T., Brown, G. and Robinson, R. (1999) 'Befriending as an intervention for chronic depression among women in an inner city.' *British Journal of Psychiatry 174*, 219–224.

Harrison, J., Barrow, S., Gask, L. and Creed, F. (1999) 'Social determinants of GHQ score by postal survey.' *Journal of Public Health Medicine 21*, 3, 283–288.

Hart, N. (1996) 'The role of the tutor in a college of further education: a comparison of skills used by personal tutors and by student counsellors when working with students in distress.' *British Journal of Guidance and Counselling 24*, 1, 83–96.

Harvey, C., Jeffreys, S., McNaught, A., Blizard, R. and King, M. (2007) 'The Camden Schizophrenia Surveys III: five-year outcome of a sample of individuals from a prevalence survey and the importance of social relationships.' *International Journal of Social Psychiatry 53,* 4, 340–356.

Hastrup, L., Van Den Berg, B. and Gyrd-Hansen, D. (2011) 'Do informal caregivers in mental illness feel more burdened? A comparative study of mental versus somatic illnesses.' *Scandinavian Journal of Public Health 39*, 598–607.

Hatchard, K. (2008) 'Disclosure of mental health.' *Work 30,* 3, 311–316.

Hawkley, L. and Cacioppo, J. (2010) 'Loneliness matters: a theoretical and empirical review of consequences and mechanisms.' *Annals of Behavioral Medicine 40*, 218–227.

Henderson, J. (2001) '"He's not my carer – he's my husband": personal and policy constructions of care in mental health.' *Journal of Social Work Practice 15*, 2, 149–159.

Hendryx, M., Green, C. and Perrin, N. (2009). 'Social support, activities, and recovery from serious mental illness: STARS study findings.' *The Journal of Behavioral Health Services and Research 36*, 3, 320–329.

Henshaw, E. and Freedman-Doan, C. (2009) 'Conceptualizing mental health care utilization using the health belief model.' *Clinical Psychology: Science and Practice 16*, 4, 420–439.

Heron, J. (1990) *Helping the Client*. London: Sage.

Heschong, L. (2003) *Windows and Offices: Worker Performance and the Indoor Environment*. Sacramento, CA: California Energy Commission.

Higher Education Funding Council (2001) *The Wider Benefits of Higher Education*. Bristol: Higher Education Funding Council.

Hixenbaugh, P., Dewart, H. and Towell, T. (2012) 'What enables students to succeed? An investigation of socio-demographic, health and student experience variables.' *Psychodynamic Practice 13*, 3, 285–301.

Horwitz, A. and Wakefield, J. (2007) *The Loss of Sadness: How Psychiatry Transformed Normal Sorrow into Depressive Disorder*. Oxford: Oxford University Press.

Houghton, F., Keane, N., Murphy, N., Houghton, S. and Dunne, C. (2010) 'Tertiary Level Students and the Mental Health Index (MHI-5) in Ireland.' *Irish Journal of Applied Social Studies 10*, 1.

Houghton, F., Keane, N., Murphy, N., Houghton, S. *et al.* (2012) 'The Brief Symptom Inventory-18 (BSI-18): norms for an Irish third-level college sample.' *The Irish Journal of Psychology 33*, 1, 43–62.

Houlston, C., Smith, P. and Jessel, J. (2011) 'The relationship between use of school-based peer support initiatives and the social and emotional well-being of bullied and non-bullied students.' *Children and Society 25*, 4, 293–305.

Howard, L., Heslin, M., Leese, M., McCrone, P. *et al.* (2010) 'Supported employment: randomised control trial.' *British Journal of Psychiatry 196*, 404–411.

Howard, L., Leese, M. and Thornicroft, G. (2000) 'Social networks and functional status in patients with psychosis.' *Acta Psychiatrica Scandinavica 102*, 5, 376–385.

Hutchinson, J. and Williams, P. (2007) 'Neuroticism, daily hassles and depressive symptoms; an examination of moderating and mediating effects.' *Personality and Individual Differences 42*, 1367–1378.

Huxley, P., Evans, S., Beresford, P., Davidson, B. and King, S. (2009) 'The principles and provisions of relationships findings from an evaluation of support, time and recovery workers in mental health services in England.' *Journal of Social Work 9*, 1, 99–117.

Huxley, P., King, S., Evans, S., Davidson, B. and Beresford, P. (2003). *No Recovery without Time and Support (or 'More than Bowling Together'): Evaluation of the Introduction of Support, Time and Recovery Workers in Three Pilot Sites.* London: Social Care Workforce Research Unit. Available at www.recoverydevon.co.uk/download/Support_Time_Recovery/STR_Worker_Pilot_Evaluation_Final_Report.pdf, accessed on 24 July 2014.

Ivory, V., Collings, S., Blakely, T. and Dew, K. (2011) 'When does neighbourhood matter? Multilevel relationships between neighbourhood social fragmentation and mental health.' *Social Science and medicine 72,* 12, 1993–2002.

Jacklin, A. and Le Riche, P. (2009) 'Reconceptualising student support: from "support" to "supportive".' *Studies in Higher Education 34,* 7, 735–749.

James, K. (2002) 'A Model of Supportive Services in Further Education.' In N. Stanley and J. Manthorpe (eds) *Students' Mental Health Needs: Problems and Responses.* London: Jessica Kingsley Publishers.

Jenkins, R. (2008) *Social Identity* (3rd edition). London: Routledge.

Jessop, D.C., Herberts, C. and Solomon, L. (2005) 'The impact of financial circumstances on student health.' *British Journal of Health Psychology 10,* 421–439.

Johnson, R., Floyd, M., Pilling, D., Boyce, M. *et al.* (2009) 'Service users' perceptions of the effective ingredients in supported employment.' *Journal of Mental Health 18,* 2, 121–128.

Johnstone, L. (2000) *Users and Abusers of Psychiatry.* London: Routledge.

Johnstone, L. (2009) 'Twenty-Five Years of Disagreeing with Psychiatry.' In J. Reynolds, R. Muston, T. Heller, J. Leach, M. McCormick, J. Wallcraft and M. Walsh (eds) *Mental Health Still Matters.* Basingstoke: Palgrave Macmillan.

Jones, I., Ahmed, N., Catty, J., McLaren, S. *et al.* (2009) 'Illness careers and continuity of care in mental health services: a qualitative study of service users and carers.' *Social Science and Medicine 69,* 4, 632–639.

Jorm, A. (2000) 'Mental health literacy.' *British Journal of Psychiatry 177,* 396–401.

Jorm, A. and Oh, E. (2009) 'Desire for social distance from people with mental disorders: a review.' *Australian and New Zealand Journal of Psychiatry 43,* 183–200.

Joseph Rowntree Foundation (2013) *Ageing Society.* York: Joseph Rowntree Foundation. Available at www.jrf.org.uk/work/ageing-society, accessed on 24 July 2014.

Kang, S. (2007) 'Disembodiment in online social interaction: impact of online chat on social support and psychosocial well-being.' *CyberPsychology and Behavior 10,* 3, 475–477.

Kant, I. (1959) *Foundations of the Metaphysics of Morals* (translated: L. Beck). New York: Bobbs-Merril.

Keenaghan, C., Sweeney, J. and McGowan, B. (2012) *Care Options for Primary Care: The Development of Best Practice Guidance on Social Prescribing for Primary Care Teams.* Sligo: Keenaghan Research and Communication. Available at www.drugsandalcohol.ie/18852/1/social-prescribing-2012.pdf, accessed on 24 July 2014.

Kidger, J., Gunnell, D., Biddle, L., Campbell, R. and Donovan, J. (2010) 'Part and parcel of teaching? Secondary school staff's views on supporting student emotional health and well-being.' *British Educational Research Journal 36,* 6, 919–935.

Kim, J. (2010) 'Neighborhood disadvantage and mental health: the role of neighborhood disorder and social relationships.' *Social Science Research 39,* 2, 260–271.

Kohn, A. (1990) *The Brighter Side of Human Nature: Altruism and Empathy in Everyday Life.* New York: Basic Books.

Kuipers, E., Onwumere, J. and Bebbington, P. (2010) 'Cognitive model of caregiving in psychosis.' *The British Journal of Psychiatry 196,* 259–265.

Laal, M. (2012) 'Benefits of lifelong learning.' *Procedia-Social and Behavioral Sciences 46,* 4268–4272.

Laing, R. and Esterson, A. (1970) *Sanity, Madness and the Family.* Harmondsworth: Pelican.

Lanctôt, N., Durand, M. J. and Corbière, M. (2012) 'The quality of work life of people with severe mental disorders working in social enterprises: a qualitative study.' *Quality of Life Research 21,* 8, 1415–1423.

Langford, K., Baek, P. and Hampson, M. (2013) *More Than Medicine: New Services for People Powered Health.* London: NESTA. Available at www.nesta.org.uk/sites/default/files/more_than_medicine.pdf, accessed on 24 July 2014.

Langos, C. (2012) 'Cyberbullying: the challenge to define.' *Cyberpsychology, Behavior, and Social Networking 15,* 6, 285–289.

Larkin, M. (2012) 'What about the Carers?' In C. Lloyd and T. Heller (eds) *Long-Term Conditions: Challenges in Health and Social Care.* London: Sage.

Lazarus, R. (1999) *Stress and Emotion: A New Synthesis.* New York: Springer.

Lazarus, R. and Folkman, S. (1984) *Stress, Appraisal and Coping,* New York, Springer.

Leach, J. (1997) *Integrating Students with Mental Health Problems into Community Education,* Oxford: Oxfordshire Community Education.

Leach, J. (2004) *Organisational Responses to Students' Mental Health Needs: Social, Psychological and Medical Perspectives* (unpublished PhD thesis). Oxford: Oxford Brookes University.

Leach, J. (2009) 'Diverse Approaches to Mental Distress.' In J. Reynolds, R. Muston, T. Heller, J. Leach, M. McCormick, J. Wallcraft and M. Walsh (eds) *Mental Health Still Matters.* Basingstoke: Palgrave Macmillan.

Leach, J. and Hall, J. (2011) 'A city-wide approach to cross-boundary working with students with mental health issues.' *Journal of Interprofessional Care 25,* 2, 138–144.

Lefley, H. (1996) *Family Caregiving in Mental Illness.* Thousand Oaks: Sage.

Lewis, L. (2012) 'The capabilities approach, adult community learning and mental health.' *Community Development Journal 47,* 4, 522–537.

Link, B. and Phelan, J. (2010) 'Labeling and Stigma.' In T. Scheid and T. Brown (eds) *A Handbook for the Study of Mental Health: Social Contexts, Theories and Systems.* Cambridge: Cambridge University Press.

Mandiberg, J. (2012) 'Commentary: the failure of social inclusion: an alternative approach through community development.' *Psychiatric Services 63*, 5, 458–460.

Mandiberg, J. and Warner, R. (2013) 'Is mainstreaming always the answer? The social and economic development of service user communities.' *The Psychiatrist, 37*, 5, 153–155.

Mankiewicz, P., Gresswell, D. and Turner, C. (2013) 'Happiness in severe mental illness: exploring subjective wellbeing of individuals with psychosis and encouraging socially inclusive multidisciplinary practice.' *Mental Health and Social Inclusion 17,* 1, 27–34.

Marmot, M. and Brunner, E. (2005) 'Cohort profile: The Whitehall II study.' *International Journal of Epidemiology 34,* 2, 251–256.

Marx, K. (1971) 'Alienated Labour.' In K. Thompson and J. Tunstall (eds) *Sociological Perspectives*. Harmondsworth: The Open University Press.

Maslow, A. (1970) *Motivation and Personality* (2nd edition). New York: Harper and Row.

Mayo, E. (2010) *Co-operative Streets: Neighbours in the UK.* Manchester: Co-operatives UK. Available at www.uk.coop/sites/storage/public/downloads/insight1_neighbourliness_0.pdf, accessed on 24 July 2014.

McCabe, A. and Davis, A. (2012) 'Community development as mental health promotion: principles, practice and outcomes.' *Community Development Journal 47,* 4, 506–521.

McFarlane, W. and Cook, W. (2007) 'Family expressed emotion prior to onset of psychosis.' *Family Process 46,* 2, 185–197.

McGowan, B. and Jowett, C. (2003) 'Promoting positive mental health through befriending.' *International Journal of Mental Health Promotion 5,* 2, 12–24.

McIntosh, E., Gillanders, D. and Rodgers, S. (2010) 'Rumination, goal linking, daily hassles and life events in major depression.' *Clinical Psychology and Psychotherapy 17,* 1, 33–43.

McLafferty, M., Mallett, J. and McCauley, V. (2012) 'Coping at university: the role of resilience, emotional intelligence, age and gender.' *Journal of Quantitative Psychological Research 1,* 1–6. Available at www.jqpr.co.uk/uploads/1/0/5/1/10511022/lafferty_2012_-_jqpr_-_coping_at_university_-_the_role_of_resilience_1.pdf, accessed on 24 July 2014.

McManus, S., Meltzer, H., Brugha, T., Bebbington, P. and Jenkins, R. (2009) *Adult Psychiatric Morbidity in England, 2007: Results of a Household Survey.* London: NHS Information Centre for Health and Social Care.

Mead, N., Lester, H., Chew-Graham, C., Gask, L. and Bower, P. (2010) 'Effects of befriending on depressive symptoms and distress: systematic review and meta-analysis.' *The British Journal of Psychiatry 196,* 2, 96–101.

Meltzer, H., Bebbington, P., Brugha, T., Farrell, M., Jenkins, R. and Lewis, G. (2000) 'The reluctance to seek help for neurotic disorders.' *Journal of Mental Health 9,* 3, 319–327.

Meltzer, H., Bebbington, P., Dennis, M., Jenkins, R., McManus, S. and Brugha, T. (2013) 'Feelings of loneliness among adults with mental disorder.' *Social Psychiatry and Psychiatric Epidemiology 48,* 1, 5–13.

Meltzer, H., Gill, B., Petticrew, M. and Hinds, K. (1995) *Psychiatric Morbidity in Private Households.* London: HMSO.

Mental Health Foundation (2011) *Learning for Life: Adult Learning, Mental Health and Wellbeing.* London: Mental Health Foundation.

Mental Health Foundation (2012) *Employment is Vital for Maintaining Good Mental Health.* London: Mental Health Foundation. Available at www.mentalhealth.org. uk/our-news/blog/120629/, accessed on 24 July 2014.

Mills, C. (1970) *The Sociological Imagination.* Harmondsworth: Pelican.

Milne, D. (1999) *Social Therapy: A Guide to Social Support Intervention for Mental Health Practitioners.* Chichester: Wiley.

Mind (2004) *Not Alone? Isolation and Mental Distress.* London: Mind.

Mind (2007) *Ecotherapy: The Green Agenda for Mental Health. Executive Summary.* London: Mind.

Mitchell, G. and Pistrang, N. (2011) 'Befriending for mental health problems: processes of helping.' *Psychology and Psychotherapy: Theory, Research and Practice 84,* 2, 151–169.

Mitchell, M., MacInnes, D. and Morrison, I. (2008) *Student Wellbeing Study.* Canterbury: Canterbury Christ Church University.

Moncrieff, J. (2009) *The Myth Of The Chemical Cure: A Critique Of Psychiatric Drug Treatment.* Basingstoke: Palgrave Macmillan.

Moore, S., Daniel, M., Gauvin, L. and Dubé, L. (2009) 'Not all social capital is good capital.' *Health and Place 15,* 4, 1071–1077.

Morris, D. and Gilchrist, A. (2011) *Communities Connected: Inclusion, Participation and Common Purpose.* London: RSA. Available at www.thersa.org/action-research-centre/community-and-public-services/connected-communities/reports/communities-connected, accessed on 24 July 2014.

Morrison, I. and Clift, S. (2006) 'Mental health promotion through supported further education: the value of Antonovsky's salutogenic model of health.' *Health Education 106,* 5 365–380.

Muhlbauer, S. (2002) 'Navigating the storm of mental illness: phases in the family's journey.' *Qualitative Health Research 12,* 8, 1076–1092.

Murayama, H., Fujiwara, Y. and Kawachi, I. (2012) 'Social capital and health: a review of prospective multilevel studies.' *Journal of Epidemiology 22,* 3, 179.

Murphy, A., Mullen, M. and Spagnolo, A. (2005) 'Enhancing individual placement and support: promoting job tenure by integrating natural supports and supported education.' *American Journal of Psychiatric Rehabilitation 8,* 1, 37–61.

Nabi, R.L., Prestin, A. and So, J. (2013) 'Facebook friends with (health) benefits? Exploring social network site use and perceptions of social support, stress, and well-being.' *Cyberpsychology, Behavior, and Social Networking 16,* 10, 721–727.

National Institute for Health and Clinical Excellence (2009) *Depression: The Management and Treatment of Depression in Adults.* London: National Institute for Health and Clinical Excellence. Available at www.nice.org.uk/nicemedia/pdf/CG90NICEguideline.pdf, accessed on 24 July 2014.

Neal, Z. (2013) *The Connected City: How Networks are Shaping the Modern Metropolis.* New York: Routledge.

Nelson, G., Lord, J. and Ochocka, J. (2001) *Shifting the Paradigm in Community Mental Health: Towards Empowerment and Community.* Toronto: University of Toronto Press.

New College Nottingham (2012) *Emotional Health and Wellbeing Support.* Nottingham: New College Nottingham. Available at www.ncn.ac.uk/content/Aboutncn/ StudentSupport/MentalHealthSupport.aspx, accessed on 24 July 2014.

Newland, J. and Furnham, A. (1999) 'Perceived availability of social support.' *Personality and Individual Differences 27*, 4, 659–663.

O'Brien, L. (2010) 'Caring in the ivory tower.' *Teaching in Higher Education 15*, 1, 109–115.

O'Callaghan, E., Turner, N., Renwick, L., Jackson, D. *et al.* (2010) 'First episode psychosis and the trail to secondary care: help-seeking and health-system delays.' *Social and Psychiatric Epidemiology 45*, 3, 381–391.

Office for National Statistics (2011) *Social Trends: Volume 41.* London: Office for National Statistics. Available at www.palgrave-journals.com/st/journal/v41/ n1/pdf/st20115a, accessed on 24 July 2014.

The Open University (2011) *Mental Healthcare Services Survey: The Results.* Milton Keynes: The Open University. Available at www.openlearn/body-mind-mental-healthcare-services-survey-the-results, accessed on 30 March 2011.

Orton-Johnson, K. (2007) 'The online student: lurking, chatting, flaming and joking.' *Sociological Research Online 12*, 6, 3. Available at www.socresonline.org. uk/12/6/3.html, accessed on 24 July 2014.

Pakenham, K. (2011) 'Caregiving tasks in caring for an adult with mental illness and associations with adjustment outcomes.' *International Journal of Behavioral Medicine 19*, 2, 186–198.

Palmer, S. (ed.) (2000) *Introduction to Counselling and Psychotherapy: The Essential Guide.* London: Sage.

Parsons, T. (1951) *The Social System.* London: Routledge and Kegan Paul.

Payton, A. (2009) 'Mental health, mental illness and psychological distress: same continuum or distinct phenomena?' *Journal of Health and Social Behaviour 50*, 2, 213–227.

Perry, B. and Pescosolido, B. (2010) 'Functional specificity in discussion networks: the influence of general and problem-specific networks on health outcomes.' *Social Networks 32*, 4, 345–357.

Phelan, J. (2002) 'Genetic bases of mental illness: a cure for stigma?' *Trends in Neurosciences 25*, 8, 430–431.

Phillips, D. (2006) *Quality of Life: Concept, Policy and Practice.* London: Routledge.

Pilgrim, D. and Rogers, A. (2005) 'Social psychiatry and sociology.' *Journal of Mental Health 14*, 4, 317–320.

Pirkis, J., Burgess, P., Hardy, J., Harris, M., Slade, T. and Johnston, A. (2010) 'Who cares? A profile of people who care for relatives with a mental disorder.' *Australian and New Zealand Journal of Psychiatry 44*, 10, 929–937.

Pollock, K. (2007) 'Maintaining face in the presentation of depression: constraining the therapeutic potential of the consultation.' *Health: An Interdisciplinary Journal for the Social Study of Health, Illness and Medicine 11*, 2, 163–180.

Porter, R. (2002) *Madness: A Brief History.* Oxford: Oxford University Press.

Prior, G. (2010) *Attitudes to Mental Illness: 2010 Research Report.* London: Office for National Statistics.

Putnam, R. (1995) 'Bowling alone: America's declining social capital.' *Journal of Democracy 6*, 1, 65–78.

Putnam, R. (2000) *Bowling Alone.* New York: Simon and Schuster.

Quinn, N. and Knifton, L. (2012) 'Positive mental attitudes: how community development principles have shaped a ten-year mental health inequalities programme in Scotland.' *Community Development Journal 47*, 4, 588–603.

Quinn, N., Wilson, A., MacIntyre, G. and Tinkin, T. (2009) '"People look at you differently": students' experiences of mental health support within higher education.' *British Journal of Guidance and Counselling 37*, 4, 405–418.

Rait, G., Walters, K., Griffin, M., Buszewicz, M., Peterson, I. and Nazareth, I. (2009) 'Recent trends in the incidence of recorded depression in primary care.' *British Journal of Psychiatry 195*, 6, 520–524.

Read, J., Mosher, L. and Bentall, R. (2004) *Models of Madness: Psychological, Social and Biological Approaches to Schizophrenia.* Hove: Brunner-Routledge.

Reininghaus, U., Morgan, C., Simpson, J., Dazzan, P. *et al.* (2008) 'Unemployment, social isolation, achievement–expectation mismatch and psychosis: findings from the ÆSOP Study.' *Social Psychiatry Psychiatric Epidemiology 43*, 9, 743–751.

Repper, J. and Perkins, R. (2003) *Social Inclusion and Recovery: A Model for Mental Health Practice.* London: Baillière Tindall.

Rice, K., Ashby, J. and Slaney, R. (1998) 'Self-esteem as a mediator between perfectionism and depression: a structural equations analysis.' *Journal of Counselling Psychology 45*, 3, 304–314.

Roberts, M., Murphy, A., Dolce, J., Spagnolo, A. *et al.* (2010) 'A study of the impact of social support development on job acquisition and retention among people with psychiatric disabilities.' *Journal of Vocational Rehabilitation 33*, 3, 203–207.

Roberts, R., Golding, J. and Towell, T. (1998) 'Student finance and mental health.' *Psychologist 11*, 10, 489–491.

Roberts, R., Golding, J., Towell, T. and Weinreb, I. (1999) 'The effects of economic circumstances on British students' mental and physical health.' *Journal of American College Health 48*, 3, 103–109.

Roberts, R., Golding, J., Towell, T., Reid, S. *et al.* (2000) 'Mental and physical health in students: the role of economic circumstances.' *British Journal of Health Psychology 5*, 3, 289–297.

Roberts, S. and Dunbar, R. (2011) 'Communication in social networks: effects of kinship, network size, and emotional closeness.' *Personal Relationships 18*, 3, 439–452.

Robotham, D. and Claire, J. (2006) 'Stress and the higher education student: a critical review of the literature.' *Journal of Further and Higher Education 30*, 2, 107–117.

Rogers, A. (1986) *Teaching Adults*. Buckingham: Open University Press.

Rogers, A. and Pilgrim, D. (2001) *Mental Health Policy in Britain* (second edition). Basingstoke: Palgrave Macmillan.

Rogers, A. and Pilgrim, D. (2005) *A Sociology of Mental Health Policy and Illness* (third edition). Maidenhead: Open University Press.

Rogers, C. (1951) *Client-Centered Therapy*. London: Constable and Company.

Rollins, A., Bond, G., Jones, A., Kukla, M. and Collins, L. (2011) 'Workplace social networks and their relationship with job outcomes and other employment characteristics for people with severe mental illness.' *Journal of Vocational Rehabilitation 35*, 3, 243–252.

Romme, E. and Escher, S. (1993) *Accepting Voices*. London: Mind.

Rowson, J., Broome, S. and Jones, A. (2010) *Connected Communities: How Social Networks Power and Sustain the Big Society*. London: RSA. Available at www.thersa.org/action-research-centre/community-and-public-services/connected-communities/reports/connected-communities-report, accessed on 24 July 2014.

Royal College of Psychiatrists (2005) *Community Mental Health Care: Council Report CR124*. London: Royal College of Psychiatrists. Available at www.rcpsych.ac.uk/files/pdfversion/cr124.pdf, accessed on 24 July 2014.

Royal College of Psychiatrists (2013) *Work and Mental Health*. London: Royal College of Psychiatrists. Available at www.rcpsych.ac.uk/usefulresources/workandmentalhealth.aspx, accessed on 24 July 2014.

Rüsch, N., Evans-Lacko, S. and Thornicroft, G. (2012) 'What is a mental illness? Public views and their effects on attitudes and disclosure.' *Australian and New Zealand Journal of Psychiatry 46*, 7, 641–650.

Russell, G. and Shaw, S. (2009) 'A study to investigate the prevalence of social anxiety in a sample of higher education students in the United Kingdom.' *Journal of Mental Health 18*, 3, 198–206.

Sainsbury Centre for Mental Health, (2009) *Delivering Job Retention Services: A Knowledge and Skills Set for Employment Advisory Services Located in Primary Care Settings*. London: Sainsbury Centre for Mental Health.

Samuel, M. (2012) 'Scotland legislates to give users right to personal budget.' *Community Care,* 1 March. Available at www.communitycare.co.uk/2012/03/01/scotland-legislates-to-give-users-right-to-personal-budget/#.UwMoPPmKWm4, accessed on 24 July 2014.

Samuel, M. (2013) 'How adult social work dealt with practice and financial challenges in 2013.' *Community Care*, 19 December. Available at www.communitycare.co.uk/2013/12/19/adult-social-work-dealt-practice-financial-challenges-2013/#.UwH-1fmKWm4, accessed on 24 July 2014.

Sani, F., Herrera, M., Wakefield, J., Boroch, O. and Gulyas, C. (2012) 'Comparing social contact and group identification as predictors of mental health.' *British Journal of Social Psychology 51,* 4, 781–790.

Scheff, T. (1999) *Being Mentally Ill: A Sociological Theory* (3rd edition). New York: Aldine De Gruyter.

Schneider, J. (2009) 'Community work: a cure for stigma and social exclusion?' *Psychiatric Bulletin 33*, 8, 281–284.

Schools Health Education Unit (2002) *Further Education Student Health and Lifestyle Survey: Summary Report for Oxfordshire Colleges.* Exeter: University of Exeter Schools Health Education Unit.

Scull, A. (1989) *Social Order/Mental Disorder.* London: Routledge.

Secker, J. (2009). 'Mental health, social exclusion and social inclusion.' *Mental Health Review Journal 14*, 4, 4–11.

Secker, J. and Membury, H. (2003) 'Promoting mental health through employment and developing healthy workplaces: the potential of natural supports at work.' *Health Education Research 18*, 2, 207–215.

Seebohm, P. and Gilchrist, A. (2008). *Connect and Include: An Exploratory Study of Community Development and Mental Health.* London: National Social Inclusion Programme.

Seebohm, P., Chaudhary, S., Boyce, M., Elkan, R., Avis, M. and Munn-Giddings, C. (2013) 'The contribution of self-help/mutual aid groups to mental well-being.' *Health and Social Care in the Community 21*, 4, 391–401.

Seebohm, P., Gilchrist, A. and Morris, D. (2012) 'Bold but balanced: how community development contributes to mental health and inclusion.' *Community Development Journal 47*, 4, 473–490.

Segrin, C. and Passalacqua, S. (2010) 'Functions of loneliness, social support, health behaviors, and stress in association with poor health.' *Health Communication 25*, 4, 312–322.

Seligman, M. (1990) *Learned Optimism: How to Change Your Mind and Your Life.* New York: Free Press.

Semmer, N., Elfering, A., Jacobshagen, N., Perrot, T., Beehr, T. and Boos, N. (2008) 'The emotional meaning of instrumental social support.' *International Journal of Stress Management 15*, 3, 235–231.

Shaw Trust (2010) *Mental Health: Still the Last Workplace Taboo?* Trowbridge: Shaw Trust.

Silk, J. (2003) 'Cooperation Without Counting: the Puzzle of Friendship.' In P. Hammerstein (ed.) *Genetic and Cultural Evolution of Cooperation.* Cambridge, MA: The MIT Press.

Simon, M. (2010) *Your Money or Your Life: Time for Both.* Stroud: Freedom Favours.

Singleton, N., Bumpstead, R., O'Brien, M., Lee, A. and Meltzer, H. (2001) *Psychiatric Morbidity Among Adults Living in Private Households 2000.* London: Office for National Statistics.

Social Exclusion Unit (2004) *Mental Health and Social Exclusion.* London: Office of the Deputy Prime Minister.

Social Perspectives Network (2014) *Social Perspectives Network.* London: Social Perspectives Network. Available at www.spn.org.uk, accessed on 24 July 2014.

SoFu (2014) *Centre for Social Futures.* Available at www.institutemh.org.uk/x-about-us-x/our-centres/centre-for-social-futures, accessed on 24 July 2014.

South, J., Higgins, T., Woodall, J. and White, S. (2008) 'Can social prescribing provide the missing link?' *Primary Health Care Research and Development 9,* 4, 310–318.

Spandler, H. (2009) 'From Social Exclusion to Inclusion?.' In J. Reynolds, R. Muston, T. Heller, J. Leach, M. McCormick, J. Wallcraft and M. Walsh (eds) *Mental Health Still Matters.* Basingstoke: Palgrave Macmillan.

Stallman, H. (2010) 'Psychological distress in university students: a comparison with general population data.' *Australian Psychologist 45,* 4, 249–257.

Stanley, N. and Manthorpe, J. (2001) 'Responding to students' mental health needs: impermeable systems and diverse users.' *Journal of Mental Health 10,* 1, 41–52.

Stanley, N. and Manthorpe, J. (2002) *Students' Mental Health Needs: Problems and Responses.* London: Jessica Kingsley Publishers.

Stanley, N., Ridley, J., Manthorpe, J., Harris, J. and Hurst, A. (2010) *Disclosing Disability: Disabled Students and Practitioners in Social Work.* Preston: University of Central Lancashire Social Care Workforce Research Unit.

Stansfeld, S. and Candy, B. (2006) 'Psychosocial work environment and mental health: a meta-analytic review.' *Scandinavian Journal of Work, Environment and Health 32,* 6, 443–462.

Stastny, P. and Lehman, P. (eds) (2007) *Alternatives Beyond Psychiatry.* Berlin: Peter Lehman Publishing.

Storr, A. (1989) *Solitude.* London: Flamingo.

Storrie, K., Ahern, K. and Tuckett, A. (2012) 'Crying in the halls: supervising students with symptoms of emotional problems in the clinical practicum.' *Teaching in Higher Education 17,* 1, 89–103.

Storrs, D. (2012) '"Keeping it real" with an emotional curriculum.' *Teaching in Higher Education 17,* 1, 1–12.

Stradling, S. (2001) 'The Psychological Effects of Student Debt.' In A. Scott, A. Lewis and S. Lea (eds) *Student Debt: The Causes and Consequences of Undergraduate Borrowing in the UK.* Bristol: Policy Press.

Summerfield, D. (2001) 'Does psychiatry stigmatise?' *Journal of the Royal Society of Medicine 94,* 3, 148–149.

Surtees. P., Wainwright, N. and Pharoah, P. (2000) *Student Mental Health, use of Services and Academic Attainment: A Report to the Review Committee of the University of Cambridge Counselling Service.* Cambridge: University of Cambridge.

Svanberg, J., Gumley, A. and Wilson, A. (2010) 'How do social firms contribute to recovery from mental illness? A qualitative study.' *Clinical Psychology and Psychotherapy 17,* 6, 482–496.

Temperley, J., Baek, P., Hampson, M. and Langford, K. (2013) *People Helping People: Peer Support that Changes Lives.* London: NESTA. Available at www.nesta.org.uk/sites/default/files/people_helping_people.pdf, accessed on 24 July 2014.

Teo, A., Choi, H. and Valenstein, M. (2013) 'Social relationships and depression: ten-year follow-up from a nationally representative study.' *PloS ONE 8,* 4, e62396. Available at www.plosone.org/article/info%3Adoi%2F10.1371%2Fjournal.pone.0062396#pone-0062396-g001, accessed on 24 July 2014.

Terrapin Bright Green (2012) *The Economics of Biophilia: Why Designing with Nature in Mind makes Financial Sense.* New York: Terrapin Bright Green.

Tessner, K., Mittal, V. and Walker, E. (2011) 'Longitudinal study of stressful life events and daily stressors amongst adolescents at high risk for psychotic disorders.' *Schizophrenia Bulletin 37*, 2, 432–441.

Tew, J. (2013) 'Recovery capital: what enables a sustainable recovery from mental health difficulties?' *European Journal of Social Work 16*, 3, 360–374.

Tew, J., Ramon, S., Slade, M., Bird, V., Melton, J. and Le Boutillier, C. (2012) 'Social factors and recovery from mental health difficulties: a review of the evidence.' *British Journal of Social Work 42,* 3, 443–460.

Tönnies, F. (1957) *Community and Society.* New York: Harper and Row.

Tudor, K. (1996) *Mental Health: Paradigms and Practice.* London: Routledge.

Turner, A., Hammond, C. Gilchrist, M. and Barlow, J. (2007) 'Coventry university students' experience of mental health problems.' *Counselling Psychology Quarterly 20*, 2, 247–252.

Turner, R. and Brown, R. (2010) 'Social support and mental health.' In T. Scheid and T. Brown (eds) *A Handbook for the Study of Mental Health: Social Contexts, Theories and Systems.* Cambridge: Cambridge University Press.

U'ren, R. (2011) *Social Perspective: The Missing Element in Mental Health Practice.* Toronto: University of Toronto Press.

Villotti, P., Corbière, M., Zaniboni, S. and Fraccaroli, F. (2012) 'Individual and environmental factors related to job satisfaction in people with severe mental illness employed in social enterprises.' *Work: A Journal of Prevention, Assessment and Rehabilitation 43*, 1, 33–41.

Vostanis, P., Humphrey, N., Fitzgerald, N., Deighton, J. and Wolpert, M. (2012) 'How do schools promote emotional well-being among their pupils? Findings from a national scoping survey of mental health provision in English schools.' *Child and Adolescent Mental Health 18*, 3 151–157.

Wakefield, J. (2010) 'Misdiagnosing normality: psychiatry's failure to address the problem of false positive diagnoses of mental disorder in a changing professional environment.' *Journal of Mental Health 19*, 4, 337–351.

Wakefield, S. and Poland, B. (2005) 'Family, friend or foe? Critical reflections on the relevance and role of social capital in health promotion and community development.' *Social Science and Medicine 60*, 12, 2819–2832.

Wallcraft, J. (2009) 'Holistic Approaches in Mental Health.' In J. Reynolds, R. Muston, T. Heller, J. Leach, M. McCormick, J. Wallcraft and M. Walsh (eds) *Mental Health Still Matters.* Basingstoke: Palgrave Macmillan.

Walsh, C., Larsen, C. and Parry, D. (2009) 'Academic tutors at the frontline of student support in a cohort of students succeeding in higher education.' *Educational Studies 35*, 4, 405–424.

Walsh, M. (2009) '(Mis)representing Mental Distress?' In J. Reynolds, R. Muston, T. Heller, J. Leach, M. McCormick, J. Wallcraft and M. Walsh (eds) *Mental Health Still Matters*. Basingstoke: Palgrave Macmillan.

Warr, P. (1987) *Work, Unemployment and Mental Health*. Oxford: Oxford University Press.

Warr, P. (2007) *Work, Happiness and Unhappiness*. New Jersey: Lawrence Erlbaum Associates.

Warwick, I., Maxwell, C., Statham, J., Aggleton, P. and Simon, A. (2008) 'Supporting mental health and emotional well-being among younger students in further education.' *Journal of Further and Higher Education 32,* 1, 1–13.

Webber, M. (2005) 'Social capital and mental health.' In J. Tew (ed.) *Social Perspectives in Mental Health*. London: Jessica Kingsley Publishers.

Webber, M., Huxley, P. and Harris, T. (2011) 'Social capital and the course of depression: six-month prospective cohort study.' *Journal of Affective Disorders 129,* 1, 149–157.

Wertheimer, A. (1997) *Images of Possibility*. London: NIACE.

Wheeler, S. and Birtle, J. (1993) *A Handbook for Personal Tutors*. Buckingham: Open University Press.

Whitehall II Study Team (2004) *Work, Stress and Health: The Whitehall II Study*. London: PCSU.

Wilcox, P., Winn, S. and Fyvie-Gauld, M. (2005) '"It was nothing to do with the university, it was just the people": the role of social support in the first-year experience of higher education.' *Studies in Higher Education 30,* 6, 707–722.

Wilkinson, R. and Pickett, K. (2009) *The Spirit Level: Why More Equal Societies Almost Always Do Better*. London: Allen Lane.

Williams, J. (2012) 'Where's the learning in lifelong participation?' *Journal of Further and Higher Education 36,* 1, 95–107.

Wolfson, M. (2001) *The Effects of Depression and Anxiety on Academic Achievement*. Nottingham: University of Nottingham.

Worral, C. and Law, C. (2009) *The North West Further Education Project: The Mental Health and Well-being of Learners aged 14–19*. London: NIACE.

Worsley, P. (ed.) (1992) *The New Introducing Sociology*. London: Penguin.

Wright, K., Haigh, K. and McKeeown, M. (2009). 'Reclaiming the Humanity in Personality Disorder.' In J. Reynolds, R. Muston, T. Heller, J. Leach, M. McCormick, J. Wallcraft and M. Walsh (eds) *Mental Health Still Matters*. Basingstoke: Palgrave Macmillan.

Young, M. and Willmott, P. (1962) *Family and Kinship in East London*. London: Pelican.

Subject Index

Author Index